HIPPOCRATES

LifeForce

superior health and longevity

HIPPOCRATES

LifeForce

superior health and longevity

Brian R. Clement, PhD, NMD, LNC
DIRECTOR OF THE HIPPOCRATES HEALTH INSTITUTE

Foreword by T. Colin Campbell, PhD
COAUTHOR OF *THE CHINA STUDY*

HEALTHY LIVING PUBLICATIONS
Summertown, Tennessee

Library of Congress Cataloging-in-Publication Data

Clement, Brian R., 1951-
    Hippocrates Lifeforce : superior health and longevity / Brian R. Clement ;
foreword by T. Colin Campbell.
        p. cm.
    Includes bibliographical references and index.
    ISBN 978-1-57067-204-0
    1. Nutrition. 2. Health. 3. Self-care, Health. I. Title.

    RA784.C5625 2007
    613—dc22   2007028580

Printed on recycled paper

The Book Publishing Co. is committed to preserving ancient forests and natural resources. We have elected to print this title on paper which is 100% postconsumer recycled and processed chlorine free. As a result of our paper choice, we have saved the following natural resources:

62 trees

2,921 lbs of solid waste

22,751 gallons of water

5,481 lbs pounds of greenhouse gases

43 million BTUs of total energy

(Paper calculations from Environmental Defense www.papercalculator.org)

We are a member of Green Press Initiative. For more information about Green Press Initiative visit: www.greenpressinitiative.org

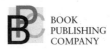 BOOK
PUBLISHING
COMPANY

 green
press
INITIATIVE

Cover and Interior Design: *Aerocraft Charter Art Service*

Printed in Canada

Published in the United States by
Healthy Living Publications
P.O. Box 99
Summertown, TN 38483
1-888-260-8458

ISBN: 978-1-57067-204-0

15 14 13 12 11 10 09 08 07   9 8 7 6 5 4 3 2 1

contents

acknowledgments

Please allow me to thank everyone who shares my life, our planet, our history, and our future. May I express my gratitude to my family, friends, and coworkers, especially those who contribute to and support the loving creation and development of this work.

I also extend my affectionate wishes to you, the readers, who by your daily commitment to yourselves and your world, enrich all of our lives.

disclaimer

The information in this book is presented for educational purposes only. It is not intended to be a substitute for the medical advice of your health care professional.

foreword

Brian Clement and I have traveled different paths to arrive at the same general conclusion about how important pure natural foods are to good health.

As an experimental researcher in the fields of nutrition and biochemistry for almost fifty years, my views have been shaped by a large body of empirical findings that demonstrate how what we eat can either keep us healthy or cause illness and disease. In my own book, *The China Study,* we presented a survey of 6,500 adults conducted over twenty years that conclusively showed a link between nutrition and ailments such as cancer, diabetes, and heart disease. My related research financed by the National Institutes of Health and published in top science journals further affirms these study findings.

During his three decades as director of the Hippocrates Health Institute, now located in Florida, Brian has seen in practice which foods are effective at strengthening the human immune system. He has worked with thousands of people suffering from every imaginable ailment. This clinical experience has enabled him to constantly refine the Institute's program of using pure "living foods" to promote health and longevity.

Having presented several lectures at Hippocrates in West Palm Beach, which enabled me to spend time with Brian sharing our ideas, I feel comfortable in recommending this book because I know Brian has substantial real-life experience to support his protocols.

Even though our views have much in common, they are not identical. (I am reminded of that old cliché that says if two people agreed on everything, one is not thinking.) My perspective on the diet and health evidence focuses on the broad and profound benefits provided by the nutritional activities of whole plant-based foods (vegetables, fruits, and cereal grains.) I emphasize the "wholeness" characteristic of food to refer to those foods found in nature during most of our evolutionary history, which have fashioned our biological responses to food.

The Hippocrates Program also emphasizes whole, plant-based food but particularizes the health effects of certain foods and food combinations by stressing the importance of consuming these foods in their raw form. From a research perspective, I only wish more empirical evidence existed for this approach using the scientific peer review process, even though that process does not always lead to correct conclusions.

Many of our most cherished traditional assumptions in the food and health sciences need much more research data. Indeed, some of these oft-cited "science" based assumptions are just plain wrong, perhaps even dangerous to the public health.

Yet, I am impressed with the significant body of evidence that points to the superior health value of raw foods. The production of toxins during the cooking of certain foods, the worrisome residues of noxious chemical contaminants in food, and the destruction and loss of important nutrients during cooking are all well documented. This information certainly supports the superior health value of raw, natural food and prompted me to conclude that if there is a better message for health than the one I espouse, it could well be the Hippocrates Program.

Like Brian, I am well aware of the hazards of wandering from mainstream science, but I also know even better the hazards of not keeping an open mind. That awareness and the wealth of supportive data for the health benefits of raw food keep me open to the possibility that a raw food diet is the most superior and health-promoting diet for the human body. If you are inclined to try a raw food diet— and there are solid reasons for you to do so—this book is a good place to start.

T. Colin Campbell, PhD

PROFESSOR OF NUTRITIONAL BIOCHEMISTRY
CORNELL UNIVERSITY

introduction

a natural healing program for everyone

Thy food will be thy remedy.

HIPPOCRATES, FIFTH CENTURY BC

Lifeforce is a power that we all possess. It is a natural and renewable resource, a principle of nature, that we were designed to use for our health and happiness. Once mindfully accessed and willfully sustained, it can extend our life-spans while giving each of us a high quality of mental and physical health.

You do not need expensive medical technology or pharmaceutical drugs to achieve this goal. Nor do you need to be a special person with superior genes in order to live longer and triumph over illness and disease. You only need to believe in yourself.

These are not claims that I make lightly, nor do I make them without the backing of a substantial body of research, as you will discover in this book. The Hippocrates Program is a collection of skills and practices that has taught at least 300,000 people who have gone through our doors how to harness the lifeforce of nature to recharge their own boundless capacity for self-healing.

Lifeforce is the inherent electrical charge from nature that regenerates human health. It is most readily accessible in raw living food. It energizes the human cell because it is the most direct connection between the sun, our most beneficial plants, and our own immune systems.

The healing quality of lifeforce springs from a synergistic interaction between our beliefs, our immune system, and the pure, life-affirming nutrients of nature contained in living food. That synergy is the foundation of the Hippocrates Lifeforce Program, and it is a prescription that anyone can master using the guidelines detailed in this book.

In an ideal world, this book would be unnecessary, because good health should be naturally occurring. But our culture has deviated rapidly and dramatically from nature's intended order. Too many of us have been persuaded by economic interests (food manufacturers, pharmaceutical companies, and medical associations) that quick fixes, magic bullets, and fortified foods are somehow a panacea for our health and dietary needs.

A direct consequence of these misguided beliefs is that we now face a chemical nightmare in our food and medicines, and in our environment, accompanied by a wide range of health challenges that have us spending more and more for less and less real care.

We are confronted every day by thousands of synthetic chemicals added to our food and absorbed from our air, water, and consumer products. Our bodies cannot recognize or assimilate most of these chemicals, and as a result, everyone alive today has become toxic to one degree or another. This is known as our "body burden," but as you will discover in this book, it is a burden that we can diminish, even if we can never completely eliminate it.

The average meal consumed today is not only laden with pesticides, preservatives, and dozens of other synthetic chemicals, it is devoid of lifeforce and mostly lacking in enzymes, the very essence of life. At every step of the food-growing and preparation chain, from crop fertilization to processing and cooking, essential nutrients are sacrificed for convenience and profit.

Our physical energy that should be used for healing and maintaining our immune system has instead been diverted to process these chemical toxins and waste products. The toxins we cannot process accumulate in our body fat and organs to become ticking time bombs. One of these bombs comes from the synergistic interactive effect of prescription drugs, which we have found at Hippocrates to be the most immediate and dangerous problem that our guests face when they first enter our program.

We can see the evidence of this toxic onslaught and the decline in our overall food quality etched in the public health statistics of countries throughout the industrialized world:

- Over a lifetime, your risk of developing cancer is one in two if you are male, and one in three if you are female. Cancer is a leading cause of death worldwide, killing 58 million people a year.
- Heart disease has become the number one killer, taking more than 700,000 lives each year in the United States alone.
- Diabetes now affects nearly 20 percent of the U.S. population. Total worldwide deaths from diabetes are projected by the World Health Organization (WHO) to rise by more than 50 percent over the next decade. Nearly half of all newly diagnosed cases will be in children.
- The WHO estimates that 1.6 billion adults on the planet are overweight and 400 million are obese. By 2015, WHO predicts that 2.3 billion people will be overweight and 700 million obese.
- It is estimated that one-third of married couples today suffer fertility problems.
- Over the past two decades, respiratory diseases increased by 160 percent among preschoolers in Europe and North America.
- Two decades ago, autism afflicted just 1 in every 2,000 schoolchildren; today autism has been reported in 1 out of every 175 children.

While all of these disturbing trends have been converging into a health care crisis, health care costs have been rising dramatically in every industrialized nation on earth. We are spending significantly more resources and receiving considerably less care.

At Hippocrates, we have seen the evidence and impact of these statistics firsthand. Over the past decade, younger and younger people are coming to us, and their health conditions are increasingly severe. We now see people in their twenties with the types of diseases that used to afflict only the elderly. We even see menopause symptoms in women who are not yet thirty years old. Girls as young as eight are entering puberty. These are the symptoms of a society in crisis.

Awareness appears to be growing that our lifestyles and health are drastically out of balance. One indication is that people feel an unprecedented depth of dissatisfaction with their health care system. An article in a 2006 issue of the *New York Times* underscored some of these concerns: "Haggles with insurance providers, conflicting findings from medical studies, and news reports of drug makers' covering up product side effects all feed their disaffection."

A result is that more people than ever before are willing to take greater responsibility for their own health. That translates into eating more nutritious foods, listening to their own body, and making health decisions "based on intuition, on our gut instinct," as several users of alternative therapies told the *Times*.

Nutrition and biochemistry professor T. Colin Campbell of Cornell University has produced more than 350 scientific papers and studies documenting the link between poor diet and poor health. His data and conclusions are unassailable. "The answer to the American health crisis is the food that each of us chooses to put in our mouths each day. It's as simple as that," he writes in *The China Study*, a book that details his landmark research on nutrition and disease. Dr. Campbell continues, "If nutrition were better understood, and prevention and natural treatments were more accepted in the medical community, we would not be pouring so many toxic, potentially lethal drugs into our bodies at the last stage of disease."

Our half century of clinical evidence gathered at Hippocrates on the health benefits of natural food, as described here in *The Hippocrates Program*, combined with Dr. Campbell's persuasive laboratory findings, present the strongest case yet for a link between toxic food and failing health, and for wholesome nutrition producing good health and radical healing.

good health is really about happiness

We often ask our guests at Hippocrates to describe their objectives for attending this program. Usually their answers are predictable: "I am here to get over a disease" or "I am here to improve my overall health." Imagine their surprise when we respond by telling them these concerns are *not* why they have chosen to participate in our program.

"You are here to find happiness," we tell them. Typically, there is a pause, and then, after a moment of reflection, the guest releases an enormous sigh of relief. Happiness is really what seeking good health is all about. To acknowledge the truth of that helps us to focus more clearly on the self-made obstructions that prevent us from achieving it.

A primary obstacle to achieving happiness and health is our doubting mind. Over a lifetime, most of us have expended vast amounts of energy creating a self-imposed maze of limitations. These limiting beliefs can stem from something as simple as an unwise or unkind criticism from someone we admired, or spring from a traumatic event in our life that shaped our outlook about whether we could trust ourselves or others.

However this belief in our limitations arose, it may be the key stumbling block to achieving the health and happiness that we desire and deserve. That is why the impact of positive and negative thoughts cannot be overlooked in designing a strategy for health, longevity, and the regeneration of the body.

A Hippocrates guest named Margaret illustrates the importance we should attach to our state of mind. She had been diagnosed with liver cancer, and after visiting two leading cancer hospitals and being told that she had only a short time to live, she arrived back home with the hope of receiving comfort from her husband of forty years. He insisted that she proceed with the suggested treatments, even though they were being described as mere postponements of her inevitable death from the disease.

Margaret chose not to accept any limitations. While under pressure and even attack and ridicule from her family and friends, she commenced a drastic change in her eating habits and lifestyle to combat the cancer. Her strategy worked. Even after her doctors pronounced her as having recovered from the disease, the skepticism about her judgment and course of action continued from most of the people in her life.

"How could you have gathered the strength to do what was appropriate for you in the face of all that resistance?" I asked Margaret. She answered by telling me a story from her childhood. Her uncle had been hit by a train and was pronounced dead. As family members carried his wooden casket into the family home, they heard sounds from inside the coffin. Margaret's father yanked open the casket's lid, and to everyone's astonishment, the uncle's sparkling eyes were staring up at Margaret.

This became one of the most significant events of Margaret's life. The lesson she drew was simple yet profound. Even in what are seemingly the most certain moments of life, such as being confronted by death, there may still be a question about whether what we think and see is really right or even real. This event inspired Margaret to always seek—and expect—a positive outcome, even when everyone else had given up hope and was arguing for life's limitations.

We all know that we need wholesome food to nourish our bodies. We also need wholesome thoughts to nourish our emotions and actions. Happiness does not mean making light of everything; it does mean learning the grace of how to live life with the bearable lightness of being.

My friend the late Norman Cousins left behind a clear and simple message about happiness and its effect on health—humor heals. Using sincere, joyous humor became the remedy that enabled him to melt away his own catastrophic disease. He wrote a famous book about the experience, *Anatomy of an Illness*, and spent the rest of his years teaching people that our choices determine whether we will create a positive or negative outcome for our health and our lives.

empowering yourself with lifeforce

Starting in 1956, the year the Hippocrates Health Institute was founded by Ann Wigmore (later joined by Viktoras Kulvinskas), we have operated on the belief that given the proper tools and environment, our bodies are self-healing and self-rejuvenating. That was a philosophy practiced by Hippocrates himself and passed down to us today from this father of modern medicine.

As a fifth-century BC Greek physician, Hippocrates treated the body as a whole, not just a series of parts, and taught a natural healing process centered on a wholesome, natural diet. He developed an oath of medical ethics that physicians today still repeat as they begin their careers in medicine. An important part of that original oath, written in 400 BC, reads, "I will give no deadly medicine to anyone."

This admonition seems to have been disregarded by much of modern medicine as physicians blindly and reflexively embrace the marketing campaign of every new pharmaceutical drug coming off industry assembly lines. They usually decide what to prescribe based on the "education" they received from the marketing representatives for the drug companies.

For a half century we have seen pass through our healing center doors practically every illness and disease known to afflict humankind. Some guests arrive after being given virtual death sentences by their medical practitioners. They are told they have only weeks or months left to live. Others come because they believe in preventive medicine, and they understand the importance of detoxifying to strengthen their immune system. Others have come to retard the aging process, control their weight, or simply enhance the quality of their lives.

People with caffeine and sugar addictions do particularly well on our program. So do people with eating disorders. If you are overweight, you will lose those excess pounds on this program. If you are underweight, you will gain pounds until your health is more robust.

You may ask how this is possible; how can the same program address such a wide range of health issues? The answer is very simple and yet has far-reaching implications. Our research has found that raw living food can trigger a safety mechanism in the human body. This food provides the body with lifeforce nourishment to bring weight back into a balance that is right for every individual. Our body receives true nourishment as our hunger is satisfied.

We believe in providing a support system so that people with health challenges can learn to empower their immune systems using the lifeforce of nutrition. A potent immune system is the basis of all physiological health and healing, yet conventional Western medicine has too often treated this engine for self-healing as an afterthought or prescribed medical practices that end up further weakening immunity with pharmaceutical toxins.

Our approach to health and healing has always been unique and, among some drug-oriented medical practitioners, controversial. But raise a mental red flag when the word "controversial" has been attached to someone or something, and watch closely for how the word is misused. Often the description of a point of view or medical practice as "controversial" is simply a convenient way for cynics to dismiss an entire body of research without having to take the time to investigate it fairly.

"Too often, controversy is not the result of legitimate scientific debate, but instead reflects the perceived need to delay and distort research results," observes Dr. Campbell, discussing how some critics have unfairly attached the word "controversial" to his own authoritative findings. "Sustaining controversy as a means of discrediting findings that cause economic or social discomfort is one of the greatest sins in science."

On a daily basis, we at Hippocrates conduct clinical research to further refine our program of nutrition and health. This "living laboratory" has pioneered research into the restorative powers of live, enzyme-rich food. After decades of conducting and applying this research, we have accumulated a vast database of knowledge.

With this book, you will reap the benefits of those many years of research findings. You will also find case studies describing the experiences of our guests who have successfully healed themselves after conventional Western medicine had given them little or no hope for recovery.

This is a self-help manual. It was designed to aid you in achieving optimum health. I will address your psychological attachment to harmful eating habits and describe strategies for you to use in creating your own support system. I will challenge you to remember that you live not only in your home, community, and environment, but perhaps even more importantly, you also live "in" your thoughts, feelings, and actions. You will need to mindfully practice what this book teaches on a daily basis to sustain good health and improve your life.

For this reason, the book begins with chapters about the power of your beliefs to shape your experiences of health and healing. Just as negativity can short-circuit wellness and recovery, positive thought can ignite, strengthen, and extend the protections afforded by our immune system. Combined with proper nutrition and other elements of the Hippocrates Program, the resulting lifeforce synergy can naturally empower and rejuvenate each of us like no other existing system of health care.

You have probably heard the expression "an ounce of prevention is worth a pound of cure." Lifeforce represents the gold standard of prevention. By embracing lifeforce and reclaiming the power to heal yourself, you will be affirming your uniqueness as a human being, and with it, your responsibility to control and navigate the course of your own life.

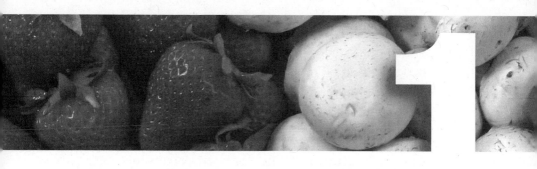

escaping fad diets and food myths

Have you ever gone through a period of trying out every new diet and weight-loss program looking for a quick fix that will work for you? Do you ever pay serious attention to advertisements in the hope of finding a supplement, drug, or fortified food that will give you a shortcut to better health without having to dramatically change your eating habits?

If you answered yes or even sometimes to either of these questions, you may have fallen prey to one of the most prevalent and dangerous health myths of our modern age—the notion that mindless eating and reflexive overconsumption carry few health consequences, and that those consequences can be remedied without altering our lifestyle choices. It is a magic-bullet fixation, and it has infected the medical profession and the food and drug industries no less than the public at large.

This state of denial about the relationship between diet and health can be found throughout the industrialized nations of the world. In 2006, a study of European consumers commissioned by Kraft, the world's second-largest food-and-beverage company, found that most

1

Europeans view obesity as a problem that only affects others (especially Americans), and they think they are somehow immune, though half of all Europeans are already overweight or obese.

A similar study in the United States, conducted by the American Obesity Association, found that 15 percent of children and teens are overweight, but only a small percentage of parents actually perceive their children as fat. "It's too painful for many parents to admit they have a fat child," commented nutritionist Marion Nestle of New York University. Half of all American parents choose to believe that their child's weight is normal.

Britain recorded the highest number of overweight people in all of Europe, with nearly 15 percent of children in that country categorized as obese. In Scotland, the situation has gotten so bad that one-third of the twelve-year-olds were found to be seriously overweight. In Australia, health authorities report that 25 percent of children in that country are overweight or obese. These countries all seem to be in a mad rush to surpass the weight problems and resulting health maladies that have been widely reported as afflicting average Americans for the past decade.

At the International Congress on Obesity held in Australia during September 2006, a statement was released on behalf of the 2,500 health experts from fifty countries calling obesity "as big a threat as global warming and bird flu." Nearly one billion people on the planet are overweight, far more than the numbers of people estimated to be undernourished, and all of this has occurred in less than one generation.

As a direct consequence of health problems caused by obesity, it is predicted that children alive today will be the first generation in history to die before their parents. "We are not just dealing with a scientific or medical problem," declared Phillip James, the British chairman of the International Obesity Task Force, which made that prediction. "We're dealing with an enormous economic problem that is going to overwhelm every medical system in the world."

No one should be surprised by these developments. Western diets now typically contain a toxic brew of synthetic chemicals that create hormonal imbalances, and those imbalances result in food addictions and chronic obesity. This conclusion comes from University of California at San Francisco professor and physician Robert Lustig, whose study of toxic and addictive foods places the blame on the food-processing industries for creating an environment that has accelerated a degeneration in the nutritional value of our food supply.

By abandoning our traditional patterns of eating in favor of synthetic, chemical-laden food—which includes processed, frozen, and fast food—industrialized nations have embarked on a vast chemical experiment in which everyone is a guinea pig. We have only to look around us at the ballooning size of people in all age groups or read the latest medical studies and surveys to see the results of that experiment on display. Obesity has been accompanied by explosive increases in the incidences of cancer, heart disease, diabetes, and an entire range of behavioral and neurological disorders.

Yet our state of denial and ignorance about these interconnections or their importance remains disturbingly high. Some celebrity role models have even intentionally sown the seeds of denial and confusion. Jay Leno, host of *The Tonight Show,* which has been the number-one-rated late-night television talk show for eleven years in the United States, was profiled in *Parade* magazine in November 2006 boasting about how he never pays attention to diet and health. "I'm a meat, chicken, potatoes, and pasta kind of guy. I eat a lot of junk food like pizza, hamburgers, and hot dogs. When I have a soda, I have a soda—not a diet soda. I don't think I've ever had a salad actually. And I don't think I've had a vegetable since 1969."

As a motivation for losing weight, people still rate looking good more important than the risk of cancer. That finding comes from a survey of four thousand people conducted in 2006 by the Cancer Research UK organization. Forty percent of the people surveyed rated vanity as the most important reason for maintaining a healthy body weight, compared to 32 percent who identified lowering the risk of cancer as the most important reason for losing excess weight.

"This research provides a real insight into the priorities many of us have when it comes to looking after our bodies and the low awareness of the link between obesity and cancer," observed Lesley Walker, director of cancer information at Cancer Research UK. Dr. Walker points out that an overwhelming volume of research has demonstrated that being obese or overweight is a leading cause of cancer in nonsmokers, and that losing excess weight is one of the most important protective measures, especially for preventing bowel, stomach, kidney, and breast cancers.

It seems remarkable that in the face of this medical evidence, our vanity can still beat cancer as a motivation for losing weight. Though this may be due in part to our biological programming to select partners who appear (at least on the surface) to be healthy, it is also a commentary on our culture's level of personal awareness and individual self-esteem. That pattern has been in place for at least a century. Our collective immaturity about health has always been ripe for exploitation by entrepreneurs and economic interests.

weight-loss illusions: a short history

- **1900.** A physician invents the passive ergotherapy chair that shoots electricity into muscles and causes them to contract one hundred times per minute. This "treatment" is supposed to cause the body to expend energy and thus shed extra pounds.
- **1910.** Phytoline weight-loss tablets enter the marketplace. They contain arsenic, caffeine, strychnine, and pokeberries, which are a laxative.
- **1914.** The Gardner Reducing Machine is introduced. To use it, a person stands between two large rollers and is pounded by the weight-loss massager.
- **1920s.** Lucky Strike cigarettes are marketed as a weight-loss strategy using the slogan "Reach for a Lucky instead of a sweet."
- **1935.** Diet pills containing dinitrophenol, a chemical used in dyes, explosives, and insecticides, are introduced. Within three years, some pill users experience blindness and even death.

During the 1950s, Americans became enamored with supermarkets and the canned and processed convenience foods they carried. The introduction of frozen TV dinners in 1954 further "revolutionized" our eating habits, and the residents of other Western countries, enthralled by everything American, soon adopted this "fast is best" model of consumerism.

As more people began to gain ever more weight from this toxic food and these toxic eating habits, a deluge of books offering competing weight-loss strategies swamped bookshelves. The Atkins Diet, popularized by Robert Atkins, promised us weight loss if we ate red meat. The Scarsdale Diet, contrived by Herman Tarnower, claimed we could lose weight if we just counted calories. The Zone Diet, pioneered by Barry Sears, advised eating five or six small meals every day. The Blood Type Diet counseled us to eat foods based on our blood type. Then came the South Beach Diet, and the list goes on and on with no end in sight.

Pharmaceutical companies got in on the diet craze with drugs like fen-phen, which was withdrawn from the market in 1997 after some users experienced heart damage. Meridia proved to be another weight-loss drug with safety concerns when it was shown to increase blood pressure. Even more diet drugs are in the research pipeline, an estimated two hundred altogether, according to the *New York Times,* and every one of them is designed to be a magic bullet that relieves users of responsibility for what they eat.

T. Colin Campbell labels this fixation on specific synthetic chemicals as a form of reductionism in science that "pins our efforts and our hopes on one isolated nutrient at a time, whether it is vitamin A to prevent cancer or vitamin E to prevent heart attacks. We oversimplify and disregard the infinite complexity of nature . . . this is not health. These are fad diets that embody the worst of medicine, science, and the popular media."

Dean Ornish and his diet became one of the few bright spots during this period because he got most of the animal food out of people's diets. Dr. Ornish also brought in meditation, which I thought was astute, because weight loss is not only about food; there is also a psychological component. His clinical studies even began to attract support from some of the big insurance companies.

But nearly every other fad diet that emerged over the past two decades has attempted to convince consumers that some combination of denatured foods can still be consumed painlessly and even beneficially. This manipulation reached new heights of absurdity during the 1990s with the introduction of almost nine hundred "low-carb" products by food-processing companies.

With all due respect to the mostly well-meaning creators of these diet programs, their complicated mazes of formulations are designed to create dietary compromises, not abundant health. Their emphasis on taste and false satisfaction rather than fuel and energy encourages poor food habits and addictions that keep us on a slippery slope headed toward illness, disease, and needlessly shortened life-spans.

What ultimately undermines all of these diets in the long run—and all the philosophies of healthful living these diets are supposedly based on—is the continued consumption of meat and/or dairy products and the absence of a comprehensive exercise plan.

We will discuss this throughout this book because it is a key finding based on a half century of research at Hippocrates, where we have assisted many thousands of people in managing and sustaining an ideal weight.

We always ask our guests if their problems stem from the food in their life or the lack of life in their food. In our experience, the answer is always both. The Hippocrates Lifeforce Program is effective at regulating weight because its primary source of nutrients is unprocessed, unheated, high-protein, living, vegetarian cuisine. Unlike commercial diets, our Lifeforce Program of living food includes the most protein-rich and least sugar-based carbohydrate cuisine in existence today.

We have found that although genetics affects everyone in some way, weight is predetermined for fewer than 1 percent of us, and even then, in most cases, it can be significantly modified. The formula is simple: eat raw, organic, living food and you will lose weight. The act of cooking—and the resultant loss of nutrients, enzymes, and oxygen—impairs our digestion and elimination, which are the two controlling factors of nutrient absorption that regulate our metabolism.

Almost everyone experiencing a weight problem can benefit simply by eliminating harmful habits. Even a modest weight loss can bestow considerable health benefits, according to Christie Ballantyne, a cardiologist with the Baylor College of Medicine in Houston, who did a study that found that a one-month decrease of just 7 percent of body fat returned blood pressure to near normal, minimized triglycerides by 40 percent, and reduced ventricular inflammation by up to one-third.

addressing the underlying issues

Fat tissue is the body's largest endocrine organ, and its volume is impressive even in people who are physically fit. A healthy, trim woman has about 30 percent body fat, whereas a healthy, trim man carries about 15 percent. The main function of these fat cells is to store excess calories. When a person becomes obese, these fat cells can swell to three times their usual size.

As obese people gain even more weight, they actually create more fat cells, which store more calories, and the cycle continues until the cumulative excess becomes deadly. All fat cells emit weight-increasing chemicals that assault every organ of the body. These cells also store synthetic chemical toxins that our bodies absorb from food, medicines, and consumer products.

Obviously, harmful food is harmful to the body; too much harmful food is worse, and too much harmful food over an extended period is usually catastrophic for health. This means that the regulation and maintenance of our ideal weight ought to be a top priority.

When people enter the Hippocrates Program, whether it is for weight management, detoxifying the body, or regenerating the immune system, the first and most important step in our program is to transform memories that undermine health. Every guest at Hippocrates receives stress management training and psychotherapy. Many of us were conditioned by our parents in ways that often proved to be mentally toxic in later life, so we work to change those memories, not erase them. We have also found that much of the nutritional education people have received is flat-out wrong. We try to counteract that with high-volume question-and-answer periods during our program.

Second, we try to make the food user-friendly. We understand the need to make food preparation psychologically acceptable, which usually means that it entails a minimum amount of time and effort. We transform incredibly nutritious food into familiar-looking dishes. This provides a gentle, toe-in-the-water approach to dietary change, rather than a cold plunge. We give people an opportunity, for instance, to make a nutritious dessert if they desire something sweet, or a wholesome dressing if they want something to pour on their salads.

A third area we focus on is movement and exercise. Diet alone does not provide enough components to build a totally healthy body. Exercise must be performed systematically and consistently. Stretching helps with posture, while aerobic exercise helps to detoxify the body. We have established that people can heal their bodies eight times faster if they do consistent aerobic exercise a minimum of thirty-five minutes five days a week. We also need to engage in resistance or bodybuilding exercises so our bones and muscles are strengthened.

The last area we address is the spiritual. We do not approach this subject in a religious, dogmatic, or sectarian way. We explain to our guests how we each carry our own burden of self, and we will do so alone unless we understand that we are part of something much bigger. Sometimes it is difficult to single-handedly summon what is necessary to get well and remain healthy. But once we realize we are part of a larger whole, it is like being plugged into a socket—we

losing weight helped me regain my health

When I came to Hippocrates, I was so severely overweight that I couldn't walk through the airport. I had to sit repeatedly in order to breathe. My entire body was wracked with pain. My lifelong obesity had caused diabetes, hypertension, and sleep apnea. I had structural damage to my body that limited my ability to even move. I arrived at Hippocrates with a failing liver, deteriorated kidneys, and a weakened spirit.

During the first week of being on the Hippocrates Program, my blood sugar dropped to within normal range, and I was able to stop taking my diabetes medication. I learned that the pain and disease in my body had an emotional component. As I allowed the wheatgrass and the nourishing raw food to support me, I began to release the emotional pain and trauma that I had been carrying in my body and spirit.

One morning, a week and a half into my stay, I was late for an appointment. I jumped out of bed, threw on my clothes, and ran outside. As I watched my feet land on the concrete, I fully expected them to break. Yet, for the first time, my legs and feet were supporting me effortlessly, and the pain that had been in my body since adolescence was gone. I ended up losing a total of 140 pounds on the Hippocrates Program. I realized that I don't have to live as a fat person anymore.

Today, my blood sugar is normal, and I take no medication. My hypertension is under control, and my body doesn't hurt. My liver and kidneys are functioning perfectly. I am fifty years old, and all of my hormone tests have come back normal. I owe my life to the program.

SUSAN RALSTON
TRUMBULL, CONNECTICUT

gain new energy and purpose. Whether you find your spirituality in nature, in quiet contemplation, or in joining a like-minded community, you can approach your life and health in a more sacred way and receive health benefits.

Being overweight or underweight is an emotional disorder. We address the emotional component and then use the tools of nutrition to rebuild the body. That is how our program works to enable people

a major lifestyle change

My fifty-ninth birthday was coming up, and I was feeling my age—forty pounds overweight, with borderline high blood pressure, high cholesterol, and questionable blood sugar. Indigestion and acid reflux made me dread eating. Worst of all, when I went for a mammogram, I was told that I had microcalcification clusters in my breasts, which could be precancerous. I promised myself that after the biopsies I would do a major lifestyle shift—regardless of the outcome.

Happily, the biopsies were benign, but I knew the calcifications were red flags. Our bodies give us signals, and if we don't pay attention, the signals become more apparent until we do. So I took the plunge and headed for a place where I knew I could do a major cleanse and diet change—the Hippocrates Health Institute.

After three weeks of eating only fresh, delicious, organic, raw living vegetables and juices, and enjoying the many therapies available, including cleansing through colonics, I felt great! Best of all, my blood work showed that my blood pressure, cholesterol, and blood sugar were in the healthy range again, and my weight had begun to drop until I lost thirty pounds. I have also kept that weight off. Even more impressive, I saw others with much worse conditions—cancer, diabetes, heart disease—begin to turn their health around. Guests came in looking gray, worn, defeated, and in pain. They left standing straight, with bright eyes, clearer skin, and a sense of hope.

JOHANNA RUCKER
TALLAHASSEE, FLORIDA

with too much weight to lose it, and how we empower people who need to gain weight to put on the pounds until they reach their optimum, healthy level. High-quality nutrients are the key to bringing the metabolism back into balance.

Our bodies can limit us or liberate us. The first step in weight regulation—whether you are trying to lose weight or gain it—is to stop counting calories and set an intention for positive change; then start keeping track of the energy levels in your food. It is the energy in raw living food that triggers our metabolism to seek an equilibrium of weight that is right for each of us.

Susan was an anorexic who, when she entered the Hippocrates Program, was 5 feet 10 inches tall but weighed only eighty-eight pounds. She literally looked like a walking skeleton. For her, the first key to health involved boosting her self-esteem. During her childhood, Susan's parents had told her that she was not as beautiful or smart as her older sister, and Susan had believed it. Once she released those imprisoning beliefs about herself, the program's diet took over, and she eventually gained forty-five healthy pounds and became a competitive athlete.

These sorts of stories are not unusual at the Hippocrates Health Institute. They are daily occurrences for ordinary people who have made extraordinary commitments to their health and healing by embracing the Lifeforce Program.

ten common food myths

Most food myths have been promulgated by food manufacturers to shield us from the truth about the impact of their products on human health. Marketing campaigns by the industrial food giants have led us to believe that specific foods are necessary to sustain human life. Here are ten of the most commonly circulated myths in industrialized countries.

myth 1
humans need to eat meat

We have been told by the meat and dairy industries that without their products we cannot obtain sufficient protein, vitamins, and minerals to sustain good health. Yet most people in Asian countries, especially China, have never consumed milk and other dairy products, and there is no evidence that their health has been adversely affected. In fact, surveys of the Chinese diet (including those detailed in *The China Study*) make it clear that the absence of meat and dairy products has been extremely beneficial to health.

Most of the world's population is largely vegetarian. In many cultures, meat is either not eaten at all or only consumed in small amounts on rare occasions. There is no convincing archaeological evidence that prehistoric humans were primarily meat eaters.

myth 2
food needs to be cooked to be digestible

This notion comes from the false belief that we should experience physical sensations during the process of digestion. That concept needs to be reversed. People with a healthy gastrointestinal tract will not notice the digestive process when they eat raw living food. However, people who have become diseased from improper diet and poor lifestyle habits *will* be aware of their digestion when they initially start eating a wholesome diet. That is actually a good sign. The nutrients in food cannot be properly assimilated unless oxygen and enzymes are present. When food is cooked, these two elements are destroyed at temperatures above 118 degrees F.

myth 3
food can be stored
to hold its nutritional value

A study done at the University of California at Davis found that a head of lettuce, once harvested, loses 50 percent of its nutrients within thirty minutes. When food is shipped, either within a country or between countries, it will often take a week or longer before it reaches consumers. This is why I emphasize the use of fresh, locally grown food whenever possible, and why I recommend growing your own sprouts. Sprouts are among the most nutritious foods available to us, and you can even grow these superfoods in your own home (see Chapter 11).

myth 4
we must consume a
wide cross-section of food

People who consume a minimal amount of food, and that food is of the highest quality, experience the least disease and a longer life-span. It is the *quality* rather than the quantity or variety of food that ensures good health. Our research leaves no doubt that fresh, raw living food provides all of the nutrients needed by the human body. An extraordinary range of appetizing and imaginative recipes have been created by chefs who specialize in raw living food, satisfying our desire for a variety of taste experiences.

myth 5
nonnutritive fluids can hydrate the body

Most beverages—from sodas to alcohol—dehydrate the body and remove the water content from cells. Only pure, clean water and fresh, organic juices can hydrate our cells. Our studies indicate that well over half of the population suffers from insufficient hydration. When we are dehydrated, our metabolism falters along with our ability to digest food; even our brain function is adversely affected.

myth 6
fruit is a health-promoting food

There are two reasons why fruit is not a healthful choice for the majority of people. The first is that most fruits are hybrids, and have been for over a millennium. In part, this hybridization was intended to achieve a greater sugar content in the fruit, making it sweeter and more palatable to consumers. There is about thirty times more fructose in the average fruit today than in the "original" varieties. When you consume fruit, you are absorbing an astonishingly high amount of sugar, which the human body cannot utilize properly.

Equally or even more important, the second problem is that all commercially harvested fruit is intentionally picked unripe. When a fruit is permitted to ripen on the vine (or tree, bush, or shrub), it will fall to the ground when the ripening is complete. This naturally ripened fruit contains all of the nutrients the human body can absorb and utilize. Unripe fruit "steals" nutrients from the human body. For example, citrus often has high amounts of calcium and other minerals when ripe; but when picked and eaten unripe, citrus drains these minerals from the body.

myth 7
we should eat a big meal at breakfast

The body's biochemistry functions similarly to a water filtration system that back flushes, except the body back flushes from eleven o'clock at night to eleven o'clock in the morning. Waste and toxins are released during this period. If you consume a heavy meal first thing in the morning, it will literally put a cork in the process of elimination. Ideally, avoid solid food at this time of day. If you are healthy, you can eat very light foods, such as juices or whole food supplements along with sprouted grains or fruit.

myth 8
if you eat a whole food diet, there is no need for supplements

After fifty years of working with both healthy and ill individuals, we at Hippocrates have discovered that almost everyone lacks some basic nutrient in his or her body. This deficiency is primarily caused by the stress and environmental toxins that are part of our modern way of life. Thus, we need more nutritional support than has ever been required in the history of our species.

We each need to measure our own nutritional deficiencies so we can choose the right food and whole food supplementation to meet our particular requirements. At the Hippocrates Health Institute, we always use this two-pronged approach to bring our guests back into nutritional balance.

myth 9
certain blood types require certain foods

The foundation of this theory is that people with certain blood types require certain foods. For example, if you have blood type O, the theory contends that your body requires some animal-based food. The Lifeforce Program at Hippocrates has nurtured people with every blood type, and we have seen absolutely no difference in healing and recovery among them.

myth 10
the Mediterranean Diet is the most healthful diet

At first glance, this diet may seem beneficial because it advocates eating a high proportion of plant foods. Pasta is certainly a better choice than animal products for promoting health and longevity. But pasta and other processed foods that are included in the Mediterranean Diet are broken down into sugars during digestion and in turn spike and then drop energy levels. Sugar in any form feeds a desire for even more sugar. Small amounts of sugar can be as harmful as small amounts of poison. If this diet consisted solely of plants, fruits, nuts, and seeds, it would resemble the Hippocrates Lifeforce Diet.

medical science findings lend support

• In a twenty-year study of over eighty-two thousand women in the United States, the risk of heart disease was 30 percent lower in participants who got their protein and fat from vegetables rather than from meat. A diet rich in vegetable protein and vegetable fat offers clear benefits to all individuals who want to cut their risk of coronary artery disease.

• Meat eaters who switched to a vegetarian or vegan diet gained less weight over a five-year period than people who made no changes in their dietary habits. A study of twenty-two thousand meat eaters, fish eaters, vegetarians, and vegans of all ages found that overall the proportion of overweight meat-and-fish eaters increased from 29 percent to 35 percent in men and from 19 percent to 24 percent in women during this five-year study.

• In a European study called EPIC involving half a million people, diet was found to be second only to smoking as a cause of cancer. Obesity was found to contribute to breast, womb, kidney, and bowel cancers, while the consumption of red meat and preserved meat was found to increase the risk of a variety of cancers.

• A large-scale study of patients with incurable lung cancer who were given just weeks to live found that "unconventional" treatments such as a diet of raw vegetables sometimes prolonged their lives or resulted in complete recovery when radiation and chemotherapy had failed to help them.

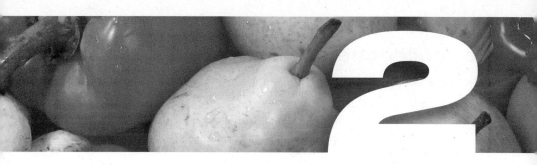

healing starts
with our beliefs

Medicine is woven into the stuff of the mind.

HIPPOCRATES

Good nutrition and sufficient exercise do not make a complete lifestyle. The people at the Hippocrates Health Institute know this and incorporate into the program a philosophy of positive thinking. The emphasis is on re-educating one's mental and emotional faculties. This seems to me to be an essential part of the strength and success of the program. Centuries-old wisdom is practiced at Hippocrates: a sound mind in a sound body.

CLAUDE BRODEUR, PhD,
PROFESSOR OF PSYCHOLOGY, UNIVERSITY OF TORONTO

Because both health and healing are so dependent on our beliefs, and our beliefs about ourselves and others are so often shaped by our conditioning, it is useful to know the extent to which we are stuck on the resistance-to-change scale. Your answers to the following questions will help to identify how prepared you are for making the necessary lifestyle changes that will bring you health, healing, and a longer life.

a reality check

1. How do you really feel about yourself?

   Your answer will reveal the amount of work that remains before you can be liberated from your own self-imposed limitations.

   ○ You feel good about yourself but want to improve.

   ○ You feel good about yourself but have several serious reservations about your ability to improve.

   ○ Your self-assessment is mostly negative.

2. Are you easily disappointed?

   Being disappointed is an indicator of negative self-evaluation. But you must also take into account that most disappointments originate from the opinions of others who are themselves caught up in their own limitations.

3. Are you quickly and severely self-critical?

   This self-destructive tendency sabotages your ability to make progress. The causes are often emotional immaturity, chronic negativity, and constant guilt. Growing beyond severe self-criticism requires powerful motivation.

4. Are you envious and resentful of others?

   When you feel insignificant, your perceptions of the achievements of others challenge you to examine your own reality.

5. Are you sedentary rather than active?

   Those who are willfully and persistently sedentary, yet have the capacity for movement, possess another form of low self-esteem. Depression often results.

6. Do you choose solitude over human interaction?

   Although solitude can be desirable and nurturing, chronic withdrawal from others may indicate fear and self-restriction.

7. Must you be the center of attention?

   Those who require constant attention live for the immediate reward. They lack the foundation for self-worth.

8. Are your relationships harmonious or tense?

   Harmonious relationships indicate some degree of inner peace. The opposite is also true. Codependency often indicates a person who lacks a core belief system.

9. Do you complete your projects promptly?

   An inability to fulfill obligations indicates a lack of self-trust. To become a responsible individual, you must establish and respect timelines, commitments, promises, and values.

10. Do you have many long-term friendships?

    Having lasting friends demonstrates constancy, consistency, loyalty, and strength of character.

11. Do you like your home, neighborhood, community, and environment?

    If you like them all, chances are high that your relationships are positive and fulfilling. If you are dissatisfied with any or all of these, it is time for a dramatic change, because we often blame our surroundings for our life deficiencies.

12. Are you willing to embrace change to achieve a happier life?

    Your affirmative response to this question is necessary for self-advancement in the Hippocrates Lifeforce Program.

changing toxic beliefs

People come to our healing center either frightened or enlightened. If they are frightened, it is usually because they feel helpless and out of control. They may be experiencing debilitating symptoms of chronic illness and they have nowhere else to turn for relief, or they may have been told by their physicians they have an incurable disease that will kill them in a matter of months or sooner.

If they come to us enlightened, having educated themselves and become convinced that the lifeforce in living food can restore them to health, they have already taken an important first step in their own self-healing process. They have realized that well-being entails more than just what we eat; it also involves our beliefs.

Harmful thought patterns can be every bit as damaging as an addictive drug. To detoxify our body we must also detoxify our mind, because our mind can sabotage even the most scientifically sound nutritional program.

We have seen this self-sabotage phenomenon frequently among our program guests. Even though they may follow the diet to the letter, their minds continue to churn out negative thoughts. They think the diet cannot work for them, or they voice cynicism about the scientific validity of the program. The net effect of this mind-body disconnect can be a disruption of the beneficial results of the Lifeforce Diet.

Your body's regenerative powers are inextricably linked to your mental state. Research has conclusively demonstrated that emotional turmoil, grief, depression, remorse, and other negative emotions depress the immune system and hamper the recuperative capacity of the body.

Altering our beliefs can have a profound effect on our lives, because what we believe about ourselves (and about the world around us) has the power to change our entire reality. Since the body is a mirror of our thoughts and beliefs, anyone interested in optimum health will recognize the value of a productive and positive belief system. And since there's no price tag on our beliefs, they could easily be the least expensive but most valuable health and fitness aid in our wellness arsenal.

Beliefs are merely thoughts that we choose to accept as truth, but if we select harmful beliefs, they can give an illness strength over us. On the other hand, positive beliefs are important to the success of any worthwhile dietary or health program, because they enable us to make progress and keep our commitments.

Imagine what would happen if a circus tightrope walker did not believe any longer that he or she could walk across to the other side. That person would be frozen in place with fear. Without positive belief, there can be no action.

A study conducted by psychologists from the University of British Columbia between 2003 and 2006 divided 220 women into four groups for math and reading comprehension tests. Two groups read an essay before their tests that claimed women were genetically inferior to men in math ability. The other two groups took their math tests without having read the essay. Guess which groups fared better in answering math questions. The women who had not been indoctrinated with the idea that they were inferior scored twice as many right answers as the ones who had been "programmed" with negative thoughts that created a self-fulfilling prophecy.

From this simple experiment we learn the formula for a positive belief system: first and foremost, believe in yourself. Everything worthwhile stems from that.

As a young boy, due to my religious upbringing, the word "belief" always seemed synonymous with fear. Every time I even heard the word, I could feel the muscles in the back of my neck tighten and my nervous system would be jolted. I eventually learned that belief is not a threatening foe; it is a friend. I now view belief as the ultimate life preserver—something that we can grab onto to steady our mind and body and bring us to a higher level of peace.

The most remarkable thing about our beliefs is that they are cumulative in their effect. The more we embrace positive thoughts and believe that they will result in positive action, the easier it becomes to maintain this outlook and create the life we desire and the happiness we deserve.

In my work with ill people, it has become extremely clear to me that those who believe they are victims, or who feel they do not have the ability to control their destiny, will inevitably go from one physical problem or disease to another until they ultimately just give up and die. Illness can be a teacher, a lesson, and a guide for us. Illness is like a tollbooth on the highway of life; it is the price we have to pay for the lifestyle errors we have made. Now is the time to let go of your past mistakes and welcome the freedom of positive choice.

the power of negative belief

How many times in your life have you seen or experienced a self-fulfilling prophecy? In my counseling work, I frequently encounter people who have created self-destructive patterns that fulfill their own worst fears and act out their toxic beliefs.

When people morosely say to me, "My father died when he was fifty years old and my mother died when she was sixty," I recognize it as an example of negative believers preparing themselves to suffer the same fate. If we believe an early death is what will happen to us, we will come to expect it, and we will actually create it.

When we were young, most of us were told that we possess some limitation, either physical or mental or both. We internalized these destructive statements, and they often come back to haunt us in adulthood.

We had a ten-year-old guest who had been diagnosed with a catastrophic disease. Her strength and unusual degree of optimism were incredible, especially given the circumstances. But the sheer desperation and pain of her grieving parents seemed to be an even greater burden for her than the disease itself. I eventually talked to her in private in my office, and this young girl spoke candidly and maturely. She admitted that her foremost problem was not her disease but her parents' fearful attitude.

She knew that her parents' concern was genuine, and she did not want to disappoint them. Unlike her parents, she believed that the disease might not take her life, and she was convinced that she could conquer it. However, her parents' lack of confidence in her survival was the very force that could undermine her belief, and with it, her ability to recover.

My subsequent conversations with her parents were an opportunity to help them develop a sense of security that would enable them to support their daughter with an optimism and confidence equal to her own. They did so, to their credit, and I am happy to report that they and their daughter are healing well together.

Modern medical diagnoses often present another opportunity for us to summon toxic thoughts from childhood. Sometimes well-meaning practitioners decide, much too hastily, that they have done everything they can for a patient, and so they end their "treatment" by declaring that the condition is incurable. Many patients simply give up on themselves at this point, which leads to a more rapid deterioration of their health, culminating in death, and thus confirming the doctor's prognosis.

A young lady came to our program a few years ago after being told by her physician that she would be dead within a matter of weeks. His exact words to her were, "Everything we have tried on you has failed. There is nothing more that we can do, so obviously there is nothing more that you can do." How refreshing it was to see this brave young woman reject her physician's death sentence. Her youthful face revealed the wisdom of the ages when she told him, "I will heal myself, and there is nothing that will stand in my way." Her hopes and her belief in herself could not be strangled by another person's imposed limitations.

"Your physician's attitude is as important to your healing as the medicine he prescribes," observes Frank Vertosick Jr., author of *When the Air Hits Your Brain*. Unfortunately, far too many patients feel impotent and never question their physician's negative opinions or judgments.

Cellular biologist Bruce Lipton's book *The Biology of Belief* documents how our positive and negative thoughts affect our cells and genes. "When a parent tells a child they are stupid, undeserving, or any other negative trait," writes Lipton, "this is downloaded as a 'fact' into the youngster's subconscious mind. These acquired beliefs constitute the 'central voice' that controls the fate of the body's cellular community. While the conscious mind may hold one's self in high regard, the more powerful unconscious mind may simultaneously engage in self-destructive behavior."

What results from negative thought is fear, and what creates negative thought is fear. The term "nocebo" is a Latin word meaning "I will harm." Nocebo is often described as a placebo's evil twin. Whereas a placebo can produce health benefits as a result of strongly held, positive beliefs, a nocebo has the opposite effect; it promotes ill health or even death from negative, fear-based beliefs.

The idea that death can be caused by a voodoo hex has been shown to be so powerful in believers that the "cursed" person often dies of fright. These physiological effects are triggered by the power of a belief. One of the first cases of such a self-fulfilling prophecy documented in medical science appeared in psychologist Dennis Coon's text *Essentials of Psychology: Exploration and Application*.

A terrified young woman was admitted to a hospital professing the belief that she was about to die. Medical tests could find no evidence of illness or disease. She confessed that a midwife had predicted that the woman's sisters would pass away on their sixteenth and twenty-first birthdays, respectively. Both sisters had indeed died on those days. The midwife had also predicted this third sister would follow them when she turned twenty-three years old. A day after being admitted to the hospital, on her twenty-third birthday, the woman was found dead in her hospital bed of unexplained "natural causes."

Research has determined that chronic stress can release the chemical messenger called cortisol from the adrenal glands. Cortisol apparently alters the numbers of immune system cells, scrambles their function, and leaves a person more vulnerable to illness. A sudden and overwhelming release of this hormone as a result of fearful beliefs may induce shock and death.

Expectations of sickness can produce sickness. A medical study done in the early 1990s found that women who expected they would one day have a heart attack were four times more likely to die from one than women with similar risk factors who did not have such a fatalistic outlook. The effects of pessimism, cynicism, and fear can decimate a person who already possesses a damaged or weakened immune system. It is a deadly combination. Fortunately for us, the nocebo has a flip side.

We have at our disposal an even more potent weapon for the healing and regeneration of lifeforce in the form of the placebo, a term derived from a Latin word meaning "I will please." A placebo is simply a belief or expectation that sparks a healing synergy between our mind and our immune system.

a husband's experience inspires belief

A year ago, when I was fifty-four, I found a lump in my throat. Concerned, I visited a top oncologist in Tel Aviv. His diagnosis of lymphoma startled and horrified me. [Lymphoma is any tumor composed of lymph tissue.]

My husband, who has been a vegetarian for several decades and adheres to the Hippocrates Program, now had a perfect opportunity to suggest that I give the lifestyle a chance for a few weeks before pursuing any radical medical procedures. So I followed his example and held to his belief that it would work.

Eight weeks after I received the shocking news, I scheduled an appointment for my second CAT scan. The doctor looked at me and asked, "What are you doing here?" He explained that my lymphoma had completely disappeared.

My husband and I were like two children in a playground. Now it's well over a year since those trying days. I am still on the Hippocrates Program, and my most recent CAT scan came back as clear as a blue sky in summer. I feel all people should give nature, faith, belief, and life a chance.

JO OLINKY
ISRAEL

the greater power of positive belief

A young woman who attended the Hippocrates Program told me about what happened after she announced her cancer diagnosis to her church group. Over the next few weeks, all 243 members of her church contacted her to say how wonderful it had been to know her. Basically, they had already given up on her survival. Imagine the impact on this young woman to have so many people wishing her a speedy death.

Thankfully, this was a very intelligent and mature young lady who realized how unproductive it was to be involved with people who had such an unenlightened state of consciousness and who had so little hope or faith in her ability to heal herself. She tuned them out and summoned her own positive belief system to start down the road to wellness.

When the founder of Hippocrates, Ann Wigmore, was told by doctors at Massachusetts General Hospital that colon cancer was going to kill her in a short time, she chose not to accept their verdict. She began applying to her life the principles that evolved into the Hippocrates Lifeforce Program. She regenerated herself until she was fully well. Her act of courage has since been duplicated hundreds of thousands of times by people who had been given a similar life-ending prognosis.

"In large measure, the history of medicine is the history of the placebo effect," writes Harvard Medical School professor Herbert Benson in his book *Timeless Healing*. Despite this time-honored tradition, Benson states, "Physicians just don't understand the placebo effect." He believes they still consider it "unscientific or a scientific anomaly."

Health continues to be viewed by many physicians as a purely biological phenomenon. But their narrow point of view is rapidly being undermined by clinical research findings that have emerged from the field of psychoneuroimmunology, a branch of medicine that deals with the influence of emotional states on immune function, particularly in relation to their effect on the onset and progression of disease. Consider the implications of the following studies:

• Measurements of the electrical activity in the brains of people using placebo pills showed distinct changes in an area of the brain associated with behavior regulation and information processing. Andrew Leuchter, author of the study and vice chairman of the

Department of Psychiatry and Biobehavioral Sciences at the David Geffen School of Medicine, UCLA, concluded that people who get well using placebos are the ones who are given hope, expectations of wellness, and encouragement. Belief activates neural pathways in the brain that influence the immune system.

• Detailed scans of brain cells in Parkinson's disease patients conducted at the University of Turin Medical School in Italy revealed that a placebo could release dopamine in the brain to ease their symptoms. "The research provides further evidence for a physiological underpinning for the placebo effect," commented Jon Stoessl, a professor and medical researcher at the University of British Columbia, who oversaw a similar study that came up with the same results.

• A study published in the *Proceedings of the National Academy of Sciences* in 2005 found that positive thinking was as powerful as a shot of morphine for relieving pain. All ten volunteer subjects in the experiment, who had their brains monitored by functional magnetic resonance imaging devices (MRIs), reduced their experience of pain by more than 28 percent on average—comparable to a dose of morphine— simply by believing they could expect lower pain levels. "Pain needs to be treated with more than just pills," concluded Robert Coghill of Wake Forest University. "The brain can powerfully shape pain, and we need to exploit its power."

As a direct result of these and other placebo studies, a notion that was previously considered heretical is taking root in some medical circles: maybe patients do not need pharmaceutical drugs after all. The science journal *Nature* raised that prospect in a 2004 study of heart patients that revealed how heart conditions were improved using placebos, which were, of course, a tiny fraction of the cost of heart medications. An article on placebos in the December 2005 *Christian Science Monitor* quoted Ted Kaptchuk, a professor at Harvard Medical School, who conceded that "most of the drugs that people take probably are not doing much more than placebos."

Cell biologist and former University of Wisconsin School of Medicine professor Bruce Lipton represents an emerging revolutionary perspective about the role our mind and beliefs play in healing our body. "When we change our perception or beliefs," observes Lipton, "we send totally different messages to our cells and reprogram their expression.

my belief system sustained me

Twenty-nine years ago I faced a breast cancer diagnosis. My medical options at the time were conventional, yet my belief system contradicted the doctor's suggestions. I had read about the Hippocrates Program and knew that it had guided people with cancer to heal themselves. This was more appealing to my husband and me, so we got on a plane and came to Hippocrates for one of the most life-changing experiences I have ever encountered.

After graduating from the program, I became devoted to the diet and the benefits increased. My children and husband had difficulty dining on raw food, so I prepared the so-called normal diet for them. My support system became Hippocrates, and whenever I needed reinforcement, I would attend the program for a short time.

Over the years, my physicians have viewed me with puzzlement. Not one of them ever showed interest in why my cancer went into total remission. Recently, my doctor at the Mayo Clinic finally said the words that I longed to hear for almost three decades, "I guess your lifestyle has healed your cancer." This is something that I clearly understood, but it was disconcerting that the people who had tended to my health could not bring themselves to understand the process of natural healing.

BETTY McCLELLAN
HOUSTON, TEXAS

The new biology reveals why people can have spontaneous remissions or recover from injuries deemed to be permanent disabilities."

Professor Lipton came to the realization that a cell's life is controlled by the physical and energetic environment and not by its genes. His contention is that our genes are simply molecular blueprints used in the construction of cells, tissues, and organs. This view contradicts genetic determinism, which is a widely accepted assumption promoted by Western medical science; this is the belief that genes control life and its destiny. Based on his research into cell biology, Lipton developed the theory that positive thoughts have a profound, positive effect on behavior and genes, but only when they are in harmony with subconscious programming. He also concluded that negative thoughts have an equally powerful but opposite effect.

So how do we reprogram our subconscious mind to positively affect cellular healing? Lipton offers two options: We can be more conscious of our negative conditioning by adopting a "mindfulness practice," similar to what Buddhists employ. Or we can alter limiting beliefs and self-sabotaging behaviors by using new "energy" modalities. He cites three programs as being effective at rapidly reprogramming the subconscious: Body Talk, Holographic Repatterning, and Psych-K.

Since our mind is such an important element in our quest for good health, training ourselves to avoid obsessing with self-indulgent and self-destructive patterns of thought is essential. Mental reconditioning that supports our health goals will be addressed in Chapters 3 and 4, where I explore the link between our mind and our immune system and discuss a range of detoxification and rejuvenation strategies that rely upon the lifeforce of pure, living food.

There is no good reason to procrastinate protecting your health. A "better" time will never come. All we have is the present, and it is only in the present that we can prepare for the future.

eight beliefs that will serve you

To make a shift from being sick (or having illness-producing thoughts) to becoming healthy requires adopting positive beliefs. Healing requires mental toughness and an outright refusal to remain trapped in negative thought patterns that undermine us. Our thoughts do indeed create our reality, or our experience of reality.

From many years of working with people who are right on the edge of giving up, we have concluded that the primary element of healing is self-responsibility. When we proceed with positive intention, we reconstitute our resources from within, tapping that deep well of healing wisdom to forge a brighter future.

Since healing begins with our beliefs, here are eight life-affirming beliefs that have become a cornerstone of the Hippocrates Program based on decades of trial and error experimentation in the field of nutrition.

belief 1: We are solar cells. The sun provides the wide spectrum of nutrients necessary for our health. Directly or indirectly, the sun provides us with vitamins, minerals, proteins, carbohydrates, oxygen, chlorophyll, phytochemicals, enzymes, and hormones, thus giving us the elements for good health.

belief 2: The three most critical foods to achieve good health are sprouts, sea vegetables, and freshwater algae. They contain the highest solar energy in the most easily digestible form available. All of the necessary building blocks for health are in these foods, in the appropriate balance.

belief 3: A diet high in raw chlorophyll delivers a continuous energy transfusion into our bloodstream, strengthening our immune system and enhancing the ability of our red blood cells to carry oxygen. The chlorophyll of a plant and the hemoglobin of a red blood cell are virtually identical in structure, making this transfusion possible.

belief 4: In the contemporary science of nutrition, the most overlooked and underrated elements have been phytochemicals, oxygen, enzymes, trace minerals, and hormones. Nutrition scientists are awakening to the importance of these factors, which are a mainstay of the Lifeforce Program.

belief 5: A primary cause of death by degenerative disease is excess protein in the modern diet. Many forms of cancer as well as heart disease, diabetes, and liver and kidney dysfunction have been linked to the overconsumption of protein. Mother's milk supports a rapidly growing baby with no more than 3 percent protein.

belief 6: Excess fat reduces the blood's ability to carry oxygen to the cells. Too often people forget that oils are a liquid form of fat.

belief 7: Much of what is available in natural food stores is not actually health promoting. This includes many of the supplements and herbal mixtures that have been touted for their healing qualities but which contain synthetic chemicals. The Hippocrates Health Institute can recommend the nutritional value of only about 10 percent of what is sold in conventional natural food stores.

belief 8: Cooking kills any lifeforce left in food. The immune system responds immediately when this lifeless food is consumed by quickly and sharply raising the white blood cell count, just as if a poison or an infection had entered your system.

You may feel some initial resistance to accepting these eight beliefs, which are the core dietary principles at the Hippocrates Health Institute. But you will find these beliefs persuasively supported by the research evidence presented throughout the remainder of this book. Once you embrace these beliefs, and once you understand the logic behind them and you begin to experience their effectiveness first-hand, you will have taken a big step in reorienting your mind to assist you in achieving your wellness goals.

results inspire greater belief

When I was born in 1942, I had a malformed left hip. As I grew, this distorted the shape and position of my legs, back, and neck, and I was always in pain. Allopathic physicians were not able to help me—in fact, they said that I would eventually need a wheelchair. A year ago, I was perusing the newspaper and saw an article about the Hippocrates Health Institute. I decided to undergo their program.

My visit was extraordinary! After all of the years of frustration, I could not believe what was happening to me. After just three days, the malformation of my left hip—which had existed for sixty-two years—began to diminish. When that happened, I began to believe more in the program, especially the wheatgrass juice therapy. I placed magnets on the most painful areas of my body, and I did three types of exercises in the pools. (Being in the water was an emotional challenge for me, because I had drowned and been pronounced dead when I was five years old! I was resuscitated, but since then I've had a terrible fear of water.)

Within one month of starting the program, the pain in my legs was gone. After a few more weeks, as I stayed on the living food diet, I was rid of all the pain in my back, hip, and neck. I now know that I will never be in a wheelchair. I am able to play with my grandchildren, ride a bike, and lead an active and wonderful life.

FLORENCE GAUDETTE
QUEBEC, CANADA

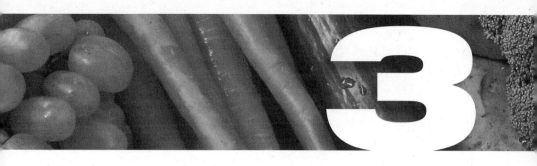

protecting ourselves from chemical body burdens

As to diseases, make a habit of two things—
to help, or at least, to do no harm.

HIPPOCRATES

We humans have become the most chemically contaminated species on the planet. As we get fatter, our bodily accumulations of synthetic chemicals increase concurrently, and that toxicity sets in motion a cellular chain reaction resulting in a greater incidence of illness and disease.

Our fat tissues are like sponges, and during the course of a normal lifetime, they absorb and store synthetic chemicals—the ones not completely excreted by our bodies, which we ingest or inhale from food, medicines, and consumer products. Since World War II, more than seventy-five thousand synthetic chemicals have been introduced to consumers, and nearly two thousand new chemical compounds are invented and added to products every year. Based on the results of research conducted on thousands of people by the U.S. Centers for Disease Control and Prevention, it is safe to say that every person in the industrialized world carries a body burden of hundreds, if not thousands, of these chemicals that persist in the environment.

It is no coincidence that during the same time this "invisible" toxic soup flooded our lives, the rates for most types of cancers skyrocketed—the incidence of skin melanoma went up by 690 percent, lung and bronchial cancer in women increased by 685 percent, prostate cancer rose by 286 percent, thyroid cancer multiplied by 258 percent, liver cancer escalated by 182 percent, brain and other nervous system cancers swelled by 136 percent. Other categories of abnormalities show similar proliferations—autism went up tenfold since the 1980s, male birth defects doubled during that same period, and infertility rose until it now afflicts 12 percent of couples of child-bearing age.

Some scientists have claimed that cigarette smoking and alcohol consumption account for most of the increased cancer rates. But that contention falls flat when we consider that an ever greater proportion of these cancers and other health problems affect children, who cannot be accused of using tobacco or alcohol to excess. What children do consume more than adults, based on their relative body sizes, are food, water, and air.

Not only that, but while children are still in their mother's womb, they are being exposed to their mother's own body burden of synthetic chemicals, many of which can severely harm a child's normal development. The Environmental Working Group, a science research organization, tested umbilical cord blood from hospitals across the United States in 2005 and found contamination by 287 toxic chemicals, at least 75 of which are known cancer-causing agents.

At the Hippocrates Health Institute, we have seen the increased incidence and severity of cancers firsthand. Several decades ago, it was rare for us to see a child with brain cancer or neurological disorders. Now we see these cases with alarming regularity.

In the Institute's early days, it was common to see elders who, through irresponsible living, had naively been destroying their immune systems for most of their lives. Back then, it usually took many decades before autoimmune diseases, cancers, and degenerative disorders began to surface and take their toll on the body. Today, these maladies erupt to destroy immune systems and health within just a few years after chemical exposure triggers the onset of cellular changes.

It is not just the individual chemical toxins that are wreaking havoc on our bodies and our health, though some of them, like the pesticide DDT (found in 99 percent of people worldwide), are virtually indestructible and present a lifetime risk for all living creatures. A far greater threat comes from mixtures of these chemicals occurring within the environment or within our bodies, especially combinations in which two or more at low levels interact to produce toxic effects more potent than any one chemical can produce on its own. The liver and kidneys—our first lines of defense against chemical toxins—are ill equipped to handle such a jumble of contaminants.

When some of these chemicals mix, they create additional chemical compounds that perpetuate an ongoing chain of new and unbridled reactions that nature cannot readily tame. Our bodies also metabolize many of these synthetic chemicals into other new compounds that transform us, quite literally, into living chemistry experiments for which there are no instruction manuals. Our very survival depends on the health of our immune system and our ability to periodically detoxify it.

At Hippocrates, we have found the synergistic effect of prescription drugs to be the most dangerous problem our guests face when they arrive. Many people take certain prescription drugs in an effort to counteract the adverse effects of other prescription drugs they take, and these chemicals combine with the hundreds of other chemicals our bodies attract to create even more dangerous combinations. Weaning our guests from their reliance on these toxins first requires challenging their belief systems, since many are not ready to give up their addictive lifestyles or their dependence on physicians, who routinely prescribe pharmaceuticals.

chemical exposure is one reason for a detox

S tudies done over the past five years by the U.S. Geological Survey and by environmental agencies in Europe have detected increasing levels of synthetic chemicals in rivers, streams, lakes, and other bodies of water throughout the industrialized world. These chemicals include pharmaceutical drugs, especially

Prozac and Ritalin, along with a wide range of chemicals from personal care products and the other conveniences of modern life.

As documented in the book *The Hundred-Year Lie: How Food and Medicine Are Destroying Your Health* by Randall Fitzgerald, these chemicals that are excreted from our bodies, or directly dumped into sewer systems, escape into the environment mostly unaltered by wastewater treatment plants, which were not designed to remove synthetic chemicals, which have been created in laboratories to be virtually indestructible. Once they are in bodies of water, these chemicals cause widespread genetic and reproductive abnormalities in fish and amphibian populations. City water purification plants, which also fail to remove most of these chemicals, draw the contaminated water back to us as drinking, cooking, and bathing water for much of the planet's population. Medical science is just now beginning to study the effects of these chemical cocktails on human health.

Given this unbridled growth in the recycling of toxins through the environment and our bodies, it is no wonder that we are the most toxic species on the planet. Here are just a few of the ways in which all of us have become human guinea pigs in the chemical experiment called modern living.

unsafe pesticide residues in food

The modern era of poisons added to our food supply came about after World War II, when the petrochemical industry created pesticides to kill bugs, fungicides to protect plants from fungus, and herbicides to prevent weeds from competing with food crops. Since that time, the levels of these contaminants in our fruits and vegetables have been high enough to inspire legitimate health concerns and spawn a thriving organic food industry. If you do not regularly eat organic food, recent revelations about the extent to which fruits and vegetables contain unsafe levels of poisons should inspire a prompt reevaluation of your eating habits.

A 1997 survey by the U.S. Department of Agriculture found that 72 percent of all fruits and vegetables produced in the United States contained detectable levels of pesticides, a total of ninety-two different pesticides altogether, including DDT, which had been banned in the United States in 1972 for being a carcinogen. In 2006, a survey of food sold in Britain, conducted by the Pesticide Action Network, detected unsafe pesticide levels between 100 to 1,600 percent above government and international safety limits. Many of these toxins are known to cause nervous system problems and other health disorders.

Male sterility has also been linked to pesticide exposure. A study published in the January 2006 issue of the science journal *Epidemiology* found the pesticide chlorpyrifos in the blood of 90 percent of the 268 males undergoing treatment for low sperm counts. This pesticide is commonly used on golf courses and on a variety of food and feed crops.

danger in our food containers

We encounter the synthetic chemical bisphenol A (BPA) everywhere in our lives. It appears in plastic food containers, baby bottles, water pipes, and medical devices, and in the corrosion-resistant resin lining of food and beverage cans.

A study published in the medical journal *Endocrinology* in late 2005 found that BPA has a toxic effect on human brain tissue. BPA disrupts important effects of estrogen in the developing brains of fetuses and children, which in turn can influence sexual development and reproductive functions. Previous studies had shown BPA to increase breast cancer cell growth.

Frederick von Staal, a biology professor at the University of Missouri, has been involved in dozens of studies of BPA, and he concludes there is a growing body of evidence that BPA can be harmful to health even at very low doses. Among the effects he has identified are alterations in hormone levels; the way the brain, thyroid, and pancreas function; and a susceptibility to obesity, type 2 diabetes, and hypertension.

toxins in soft drinks

Tests conducted on 230 soft drink brands sold in Britain and France found benzene levels eight times higher than the allowable level in drinking water, according to a 2006 report by Britain's Food Standards Agency. Benzene is produced from petrochemicals and is used as an engine antiknock agent in gasoline.

Benzene toxicity has been linked to leukemia and other cancers of the blood. Some food scientists believe the benzene in soft drinks may have been produced by a reaction of two chemical ingredients used in manufacturing soft drinks: the preservative sodium benzoate and ascorbic acid.

mercury poisoning moves beyond fish

We have heard about high levels of mercury contaminating certain types of ocean fish, such as tuna and swordfish, which has resulted in health advisories for pregnant women and children. Now the concerns have shifted to a type of mercury contamination that is not so easily avoided.

Coal-burning power plants, wastewater treatment plants, and waste incinerators have been spewing out tons of mercury into the environment, and this pollution is affecting the reproduction and behaviors of both freshwater fish and wildlife. A 2006 report by the National Wildlife Federation in the United States concluded that every aspect of our food web and ecosystem has been contaminated—from ocean to forest to coastal waters to wetlands. Mercury toxicity bioaccumulates up the food chain, and humans are at the top of that chain.

a Teflon chemical pollutes us all

Out of 300 umbilical cords from newborn babies tested by researchers at Johns Hopkins Hospital in Baltimore, 298 of them contained a suspected carcinogenic chemical used to make Teflon, the coating on nonstick cookware. How it got into the bloodstreams of mothers and infants "is a mystery," said Frank Witter, medical director of labor and delivery at the Johns Hopkins School of Medicine and a partner in the research, when the study results were released in February 2006.

Previous testing had detected the chemical, called perfluorooctanoic acid (PFOA), in the bodies of most adults in industrialized countries. It has even been measured in the flesh and blood of polar bears in the Arctic region. Scientists speculate that it is released during the manufacturing process and migrates through air and water—its molecules attached to dust particles—until it lodges in whatever lifeform happens to absorb it. It may also enter the body from contact with the many types of consumer products—such as microwave popcorn bags—that contain it. While DuPont, the sole North American producer of PFOA, continues to maintain that the chemical poses no danger to human health, studies are accumulating that indicate PFOA can alter human hormone levels and cause birth defects.

In early February 2006, the U.S. Environmental Protection Agency Science Advisory Board voted unanimously that PFOA should be labeled "a likely carcinogen." The EPA urged DuPont to eliminate this chemical from its production process by the year 2015, which means we still have many years of continued PFOA production and use before this worldwide experiment on us and our children finally comes to an end.

consumer product chemicals in food

A European environmental group called WWF (formerly known as the World Wildlife Fund) tested twenty-seven foods commonly sold in supermarkets throughout the seven European Union countries and discovered every single item was contaminated with chemicals from ordinary consumer products. This 2006 study of meat, fish, bread, olive oil, and dairy products looked for such man-made chemicals as PCBs, brominated flame retardants, perfluorinated chemicals, phthalates, artificial musks, and pesticides. Every food sample contained some or most of these chemicals. "Nowhere near enough is known about the long-term effects of exposure to multiple chemical contaminations," remarked Paul King, director for WWF-UK. Over long periods of time, the food we eat contributes significantly to our body burden of chemicals.

synthetics can cause brain disorders

By some estimates, one in every six of the world's children suffers a developmental disability such as autism, cerebral palsy, or attention deficit disorder. The primary culprits, according to researchers at the Harvard University School of Public Health, are 202 synthetic chemicals that can be harmful to humans even at low levels of exposure. These chemicals can be found in many household products ranging from styrene in plastics to the aluminum in soda cans and acetone in nail polish remover. Later in life, this cumulative chemical exposure may trigger Parkinson's disease and other neurological disorders.

chemical harm can be inherited

One of the more disturbing developments over the past few years was the discovery that environmental influences—especially chemical harm—can be passed on to our children and grandchildren as a modification to their genes. Previously, it had been thought that parents can only pass potential health problems to their offspring as a result of genetic mutations. This latest research, pioneered by biologists at Washington State University in 2005, found that a pregnant woman who is exposed to a pesticide or any other chemical toxin can transfer the damage or disease caused by the toxin to her children, grandchildren, and all future descendants, without changes in her own genetic code. Rather than an alteration in DNA sequence, it is a chemical modification of the DNA that can be inherited, a process that has been labeled "epigenetic change." The implications of this finding for public health are enormous. Within a year of this research being publicized, another team of researchers at Vanderbilt University discovered that a change in one gene's expression, as might be caused by a mother's exposure to a synthetic chemical toxin, can be the environmental trigger that results in a child developing autism. Many more health outcomes for future generations are being programmed into the human fetus than scientists ever previously thought possible.

removing toxins
that degrade lifeforce

We ask every guest coming to Hippocrates to arrive without any synthetic chemicals in their possession, especially in their personal care products. Their first step in the healing process is to remove as many toxins from their body as possible to allow the organs and immune system to operate most efficiently. These toxins are most often embedded in the cell structure of the body, so we must rebuild the body to introduce healthy cells to regenerate health, and that means first initiating a detoxification regimen.

All of us should consider undergoing detoxification as a process for maintaining health. A juice fast one day a week would be helpful. Exercise, colon cleanses, and eating pure, natural, organic food also help. Having a detox strategy for yourself and those you love is a survival mechanism that can help to maintain good health and maybe even prevent premature death.

Each aspect of the detox program is equally important. If you are constipated, colon cleansing should be your first step. If you have poor digestion or you have a cold, fasting might be the most important first step. Exercise that works up a sweat can effectively remove some toxins from the body via perspiration.

As far as supplements, chlorella is at the top of the list for detox. It is the most effective of the green algae in taking out heavy metals and radiation from the body, as it has a mineral complex that magnetizes toxins and acts as a sponge to soak them up. When my wife and I were in Russia, we used a combination of chlorella and chlorophyll to help rid radioactivity from people who were exposed to it during the Chernobyl disaster. Russian research scientists told us this proved to be the most effective detox.

Following chlorella on the list of important detoxifiers is capsicum, the extract of cayenne pepper, which increases circulation and warms up the body, causing us to perspire. Capsicum positively influences cardiovascular health.

detoxification yields unexpected benefits

Having been an Olympic gymnast and recreational athlete, I have always been conscious about my body and my overall health. Over the last twenty years, I have often chosen to spend my vacations at health spas. Hippocrates turned out to be much more than a health spa. My experience at this unique healing institute surpassed all my expectations.

My primary goal in attending the program was to learn how to thoroughly detoxify my body, purify my mind, and transform the quality of my life. At first I found it overwhelming, and the lifestyle changes were challenging. But as I immersed myself fully in the wheatgrass and juice therapies, organic living food, colon cleanses, far-infrared sauna, exercise, and other detox therapies, it became much easier.

At the end of three weeks, I felt energized, empowered, and transformed. Since then, my eyesight has improved, and I find that it is much easier to maintain my ideal weight. My participation in the Hippocrates Program was one of the most rewarding experiences of my life, equivalent to my participation as a gymnast in the XIV Olympiad in London in 1948.

ROSE VOISK
NEW YORK

Garlic is next on the list, as it is most effective at killing microbes and eliminating them from the body. It also helps rid the body of mold and fungi. Edible green clay can be effective in ridding the body of poisons. Equally important is consuming large amounts of organic cruciferous vegetables, because the sulfur they contain can attract and remove poisons and mutagens from the system.

the role of fasting

Throughout human history, fasting has been recognized in numerous cultures as an important practice for eliminating toxins from the body. Many historical figures in the Bible regularly fasted. In more recent times, Gandhi, Martin Luther King Jr., and Mother Teresa were among those who engaged in this healing practice.

Two schools of thought have emerged about food abstinence. One point of view holds that water fasts are the only correct way, while another view suggests that fasting can and should include organic plant juices for the best results. At Hippocrates, we subscribe to the latter view.

We have found that although drinking water by itself can greatly accelerate the release of toxins from the body, water fasting alone can cause unnecessary stress on the organs of elimination. Juice fasting

TABLE 1: *a sample fasting plan*

TIME OF DAY	JUICE OPTIONS
Before breakfast	2 ounces wheatgrass juice
Breakfast	16 ounces green vegetable juice or green drink consisting of vegetables, such as celery, cucumbers, summer squash, parsley, watercress, and sprouts (sunflower, mung bean, green pea, clover, and/or fenugreek)
Lunch	16 ounces sprout juice, green vegetable juice, or a mixture of green vegetable juice, fruit juice, and/or pure water
Bedtime	2 ounces wheatgrass juice
Between-meal snacks and drinks	16 ounces green vegetable juice, extremely diluted fruit juices (for those who are not concerned about their sugar intake), or lemon water sweetened with stevia

can be just as effective as water and simultaneously nourishes and strengthens the body rather than depleting and weakening it.

Green juices and wheatgrass juice are the fasting nourishments of choice at Hippocrates. These vital juices offer the body complete proteins, which help to regulate blood sugar, and provide enzymes, which provoke emulsification of particulate matter in the organs of the body. They also supply oxygen, which acts as an antiseptic and metabolism regulator. Fasting on these green drinks affords the body greater detoxification with less discomfort than purified water alone.

Fasting can be good for everyone, with these exceptions: do not fast if you have a blood sugar disorder and you are gaunt, weak, or impaired in any other way (including emotionally). If you are considering a fast, first consult a health practitioner, such as a naturopathic physician, who is open-minded about the procedure and qualified to advise you.

We recommend fasting for twenty-four hours once a week. Table 1 provides an example of a good fasting plan. Please note that all water must be pure, either molecularly organized or distilled, and that all food you'll be using to make your juices must be organically grown. Wheatgrass juice accelerates detoxification and is an unsurpassed blood purifier and blood strengthener. It is rich in chlorophyll, essential amino acids, vitamins A and C, sulfur, phosphorus, and the minerals calcium, iron, and zinc.

the role of colon hydrotherapy

Our body's large intestine is the channel for eliminating solid waste. After years of chemical exposure and processing low-enzyme and low-quality food, the colon weakens and the accumulation of waste along the colon's walls gradually attracts the growth of unfriendly bacteria that feed off the stagnant waste material. This forms an unhealthy colon and creates symptoms of physical toxicity.

Our program's colon cleanses involve the use of enemas and colonic irrigation treatments that utilize wheatgrass or algae implants. During decades of research at Hippocrates, we have found that this practice helps to restore the electrolyte and mineral balance in the colon while cleansing the system of toxins.

Cleansing the colon with water dates from ancient times, and some Western hospitals continued the practice until the 1940s. Many elderly physicians have told me stories about the vast health benefits colon irrigation afforded their patients and how, on occasion, the practice even eliminated the need for radical medical procedures and surgeries.

Modern colonics have evolved into a gentle and comfortable procedure that has proven simple, safe, and effective in loosening and dissolving impurities from the walls of the colon. This waste matter, if not periodically removed, putrefies through bacterial action to make the colon sluggish and toxic.

the role of lymphatic drainage massage

This body-massage technique assists the flow of lymph along its normal glandular routes. The goal is to reduce congestion and the retention of wastes and strengthen the immune system.

Impairment of the lymphatic system flow can stem from infection, poor diet, stress, shallow breathing, and/or a lack of proper exercise. Lymphatic drainage massage, in our experience, has proven effective against illnesses and disorders specific to the lymphatic system. It is also a beneficial treatment or adjunctive therapy for any condition that makes demands on the body's defense system.

During an internal program review study conducted at Hippocrates in 1981, we gave twice weekly massages for a month to seventy-eight people and compared their levels of liver and gallbladder enzymes to seventy-eight other people who received no bodywork during that period. The people who received the detox massages showed a 35 percent increase in enzyme regulation. That finding was important, because when people have toxins in their system, blood tests reveal the effects on the levels of enzymes in their liver and gallbladder. Therapeutic massage helps to regulate enzymes and move them into a healthier range, thereby assisting the body in removing toxins.

A second internal program review study in 1982 placed ninety people on supplemental digestive enzymes. We found a connection between this enzyme supplementation and cholesterol reduction. As we increased the amounts of enzymes they took, we discovered that particulate pollutants stored in body fat were greatly reduced.

the role of physical exercise

Vigorous physical activity is one of the human body's greatest allies in the fight against environmental toxicity. When we exercise, our lymphatic and respiration systems, which include the lungs and the skin (our largest body organ), release some of the chemicals we absorb on a daily basis, which our body stores.

When we are inactive due to lethargy, obesity, depression, or force of habit, these accumulated chemicals stagnate in our cells. Both children and adults are much less physically active than people were just a generation ago, yet we are exposed to ten times more synthetic chemical toxins.

Our bloodstream carries nutrients, which are extracted from the food we eat, to every cell in our body. Exercise facilitates the journey of these nutrients while generating enormous amounts of oxygen in the bloodstream. This highly oxygenated blood helps the nutrients that constitute our fuel to be burned more readily. Exercise quite literally nourishes our cells.

Our bloodstream is also a sanitation department, clearing our systems of any residue that remains after the food fuel has been burned. Vigorous exercise helps the bloodstream to perform that role more efficiently. Finally, an unimpeded bloodstream keeps our veins and arteries open, which inhibits the accumulation of cholesterol.

the role of far-infrared saunas

A relatively recent but important component of our detox program involves the use of far-infrared saunas, which produce high energy as opposed to the high heat of conventional saunas. Far-infrared energy safely penetrates at least three inches into body tissues to help release chemical toxins that regular saunas fail to reach and excrete.

One of our guests for three weeks in late 2005 was investigative journalist Randall Fitzgerald, the author of *The Hundred-Year Lie*, who used our detox program for his own experiment to test how quickly and thoroughly synthetic chemicals could be leached from his body. His blood was drawn and tested by a laboratory in Dallas, Texas, and the report came back showing that he had the usual body burden of hundreds of chemicals that we all carry, but he had particularly high levels of DDE (a breakdown component of DDT) and mirex, an ant killer.

Fitzgerald followed the same detoxification program as all our guests—drinking wheatgrass juice, eating raw living food, fasting for a day once a week, and doing a weekly colonic. He did daily cardio

purging toxins rejuvenated health

F or many years I had been suffering from candidiasis without knowing it or recognizing its vague symptoms. I had a rash all over my hands, arms, and legs. My abdomen was distended so much that I looked like I was in my seventh month of pregnancy. I was taking medication for asthmalike symptoms, as the fungus had spread into my lungs and was causing breathing problems.

By compromising my immune system, candidiasis made me vulnerable to a host of other problems, including polio and leukemia. My arduous search for good health led me to the Hippocrates Program. I spent three weeks in intensive detoxification. After the three weeks, my rash gradually disappeared, and my abdomen deflated to one-quarter of its bloated size. I began to feel as if a heavy load had been lifted off of me. I was told this was the result of toxins being eliminated from my body. My white hair has even returned to its original brown color. I am finally back to good health, and I am continuing to adhere to this remarkable program.

PATRICIA WILLIAMS
WEST PALM BEACH, FLORIDA

exercise followed by fifteen minutes in the far-infrared sauna. He also took chlorella supplements, which contain a freshwater alga that aids in the removal of chemicals from the body.

After three weeks on the Lifeforce Program, he had his blood tested again by the same laboratory. Both the laboratory and Fitzgerald found the test results to be stunning. The chief toxicologist and laboratory director, John Laseter, reported that Fitzgerald had reduced the levels of DDE and mirex in his body by two-thirds. Levels of other chemical toxins also fell dramatically, which meant his body fat and organs were releasing toxins that ordinarily might have taken much longer to excrete, if they were excreted at all.

Sweating out toxins has a rich historical tradition. Whether it was sweat lodges in American Indian cultures, the saunas popularized in Nordic cultures, or Turkish steam baths, people have long understood the benefits of detoxifying the body. Modern Western medicine is finally beginning to embrace the idea that hyperthermia can boost the immune system as it detoxifies the body.

the role of pure water

Like the battery in your car, your cells are responsible for charging you up with energy and vitality. When you feel lifeless, you are suffering from a lack of vital energy, much like a stalled car. Since every body is in essence a rechargeable vehicle, it can be reinvigorated to run smoothly and efficiently; it just takes the right fuel and constant care. The second most important element of life itself, after oxygen, is pure water.

Water is the primary conductor of the body's electric current, and our cells require pure water on a regular basis. Water that is full of impurities and biologically incompatible chemicals prevents the constructive interaction of bodily systems and encourages cancer-causing activity.

Pure water is an unrestricted highway on which all intercellular activity moves freely. This unrestricted flow allows the meridian system, the body's electrical roadway, to stay fully charged at all times, creating a powerful, protective shield that prevents free radicals (reactive atoms that are produced in the body and can damage cells, proteins, and DNA by altering their chemical structure) from destroying healthy cells. Free radical damage is the cause of disease, premature aging, and all the body's internal plagues.

The natural metabolic processes of the body—including digestion and elimination—create toxic by-products. Because the production of these by-products is a perfectly normal function, they occur even in those who follow the Hippocrates Lifeforce Program. Exercise encourages perspiration and the flow of blood, which cleanse the respiratory and circulatory systems of particulates that stifle systematic electrical functioning. Eliminating poisons from the body allows greater absorption of nutrients and accelerates all healthy body functions.

Hormones, the chemical messengers of the body, flourish in a clean bloodstream, because the communication between cells, tissues, and organs requires a constantly clear channel. Many kinds of brain disorders and body malfunctions occur because of a hormonal imbalance often caused by the absence of clear cell-to-cell directives. Thyroid dysfunction, which is increasing worldwide at alarming rates, has a profound impact on our minds and metabolism. In many people, the pituitary gland, at the center of the brain, is apparently dysfunctional. This core of hormonal generation empowers other

a detox to relieve asthma

Over a period of two and a half years, my health started to decline. I had high blood pressure and high cholesterol and had been on medication for asthma since my diagnosis in 1990. The coughing associated with my asthma had always been very embarrassing for me, but my biggest fear was that someday my asthma would get so bad I would have to be on oxygen like my mother had been.

I had visited more than ten doctors, seeking relief for the persistent pain in my neck, shoulders, knees, and feet. Every doctor came up with a different diagnosis for this chronic joint pain. I heard so many different opinions that I was confused and overwhelmed, and I became depressed.

Someone had given my husband *The China Study* by T. Colin Campbell, and the book piqued my interest. For about three months, I tried following the plan outlined in the book; it helped with the chronic pain but had no effect on my asthma. Then I learned about the Hippocrates Program and decided to try it.

When I arrived, I was surprised at how willingly I embraced the program. I knew immediately I was where I needed to be. After three weeks of detox and a living food diet, I had lost nineteen pounds and my blood pressure had returned to normal without medication. My cholesterol went from 256 to 192! It is now seven months later, and I continue to be completely off all my asthma medication and all prescription drugs. I am happy, my energy level is high, and my days and nights are free of pain.

VICKY ANTHONY
SOUTH CAROLINA

glands, so when it produces either too few or too many hormones, all other glands and their anatomical connections malfunction and degenerate—sometimes permanently. Electrochemical charge, the foundation of functional life, must be constantly renewed—with the assistance of abundant pure water—otherwise, our health, emotions, thoughts, spirit, rest, functioning, and movement all suffer.

Here are three tips for success in keeping the water that enters your body pure:

1. Do not drink tap water provided by local governments. Not only does most of it contain harmful levels of chlorine and fluoride, it is also contaminated with a wide range of synthetic chemical toxins that water purification plants cannot remove.

2. Do not drink most bottled water. Many brands, such as Aquafina and Dasani, the two best-selling brands in the United States, are just municipal tap water that has been crudely filtered.

3. Purchase your own high-quality charcoal water filters and use them for all of the water you consume.

the role of wheatgrass juice

Studies have found that wheatgrass juice is almost pure chlorophyll, and chlorophyll functions similarly to red blood cells, thus helping to clean out our arteries. The nutrients and oxygen that chlorophyll naturally contains help to flush out toxins from the human body while stimulating bone marrow to produce new cells.

Wheatgrass juice is the core reason why the Hippocrates Program has been so effective at regenerating the human body. The foods with the highest chlorophyll content also have the highest amount of phytochemicals, which aid in protecting us against disease. Of all these foods, sprouted wheatgrass has the highest content of both chlorophyll and phytochemicals.

Two scientists with the Department of Physiology at the University of Liverpool induced anemia in two groups of rabbits and then tested them to determine the ability of chlorophyll to regenerate their blood. The first group received chlorophyll in their daily diet, while the second group did not. The animals in the first group were able to convert the chlorophyll into new blood cells and overcome their anemia, but the second group remained severely anemic.

A complete and total detoxification of the body can take up to seven years, the same period of time it takes for us to replace all of the cells in our body. More than half of the accumulated wastes in our body will be released the first seven days of a detox program, but complete healing and restoration of the body can be broken down into stages, as outlined in Table 2.

TABLE 2: *stages of detoxification*

NUMBER OF YEARS AFTER DETOX	RESULTS
Up to 1½ years	Major digestive cleansing with removal of fat deposits and calcifications
1½ to 2 years	Deep tissue and joint cleansing
2 to 5 years	Bone structure, cartilage, and further joint cleansing
5½ to 6 years	Organ repositioning and renewal
6 to 7 years	Brain tissue and neurological cleansing

As layer after layer of contaminants are stripped away, the release of toxins will periodically affect how you feel. But as time passes, your overall health and feelings of wellness will markedly improve. Due to the body's cellular intelligence, every part is affected by the whole. When one part of us is renewed, our entire body benefits from greater harmony and integration.

4

nature's gift
to our health

*The natural healing force within each one of us
is the greatest force in getting well.*

HIPPOCRATES

We each have within us an extraordinary mechanism for self-healing. It is that community of highly specialized cells that we call our immune system, which can be regenerated as needed using the lifeforce of nature.

When functioning properly, this inner healing clinic of over two trillion defenders is capable of identifying and eliminating alien invaders that threaten our health and our lives. The T cells, H cells, and leukocytes (white blood cells) that constitute the core elements of this system perform unique roles that require our nutritional support and ongoing detoxification of the body.

An average five-year-old child who comes inside the house covered in grime after a day of playing outside is under attack by thousands of various viruses, bacteria, protozoa, fungi, and other microbes. The child's armor of skin cells captures many of these microbes, which are then dispatched as the skin cells undergo normal shedding. The child's eyes are naturally cleansed with continuous blinking that summons antiseptic fluid from the tear ducts. Meanwhile, the mucus in the child's nostrils are trapping airborne toxic invaders. Acids in the stomach and immune cells in the intestinal tract are attacking microbes that live on the food the child has ingested. The immune system is also identifying and destroying mutant cells within the body that could cause cancer.

When the body detects invaders, immune cells release chemicals called interferon and interleukins, which mobilize many other immune system warriors to play various roles. Proteins called immunoglobulins are sent out like scouts to investigate. If these immunoglobulins determine that the body is under assault from cancers, viruses, or other microbes, the body activates T cells and other "killer" cells to be the soldiers that destroy these unwelcome visitors.

Never before in human history have our immune systems been under such a systematic and sustained assault as we face today. Synthetic chemical toxins in our air, water, food, medicines, and consumer products are the new threats that combine with the microbes we have always faced, yet now these toxins have multiplied by the hundreds of thousands to weaken our immunity to illness and disease. Add toxic thoughts to this noxious stew and we have the ingredients for an immune system breakdown.

Imagine the effect on us if we had to work nonstop at a job twenty-four hours a day, seven days a week. That is what the stresses of modern life are putting our immune systems through, and the strain often leads to premature exhaustion, aging, and disease.

One of the symptoms of this immune system exhaustion—and the resulting increased vulnerability to disease—can be seen in the numbers of people who are unknowingly infested with *Candida albicans,* a yeastlike fungus that is found naturally almost everywhere in our external environment. Once this fungus invades the human body, our cells become deoxygenated.

In chronic candidiasis, the yeast invades organ tissues, such as the lungs and liver, creating even more serious health problems. It is an opportunistic microbe that takes advantage of weakened immune systems. Consequently, when a person is facing cancer, diabetes, cardiovascular illness, and other such health challenges, *Candida albicans* may also be present, posing additional roadblocks to recovery.

Candida is closely related to hypoglycemia and diabetes, because this yeast infestation actually draws blood sugar to feed itself. If you are experiencing any symptoms of hypoglycemia, it is important to recognize that your susceptibility to *Candida* is greatly increased. Some symptoms of moderate *Candida* are itchy nose and eyes, nasal drip, a congested throat, fatigue, and a generally confused state of mind.

Several prescription drugs are commonly touted as remedies for *Candida*, but we have observed that these drugs act to further weaken the immune system. Probably the worst solution for *Candida* offered up by some medical "authorities" is for the sufferer to consume more animal products. Based on our observations, research, and findings at Hippocrates, this approach simply exacerbates and perpetuates the problem. Imagine the internal body, once infected with *Candida*, as a dank, moldy, dripping cave; this paints a rather accurate picture of what is going on inside.

If you have an enzyme-deficient diet and your tissues are oxygen starved, you have unwittingly created an ideal environment for this fungus to prosper. The most effective way to clean up and rejuvenate the affected internal areas is to expose the body to various forms of sunlight and air. This means eating a diet of raw, unprocessed vegetables and germinated seeds, grains, nuts, and beans, which transfer sunlight energy—the lifeforce—to clean up our cellular environment. Combine this with a regular exercise program, preferably out-of-doors, and the *Candida* problem will be alleviated.

The potential for our diets to boost our immune system is directly linked to the quality of the soil in which our food is grown. Soil depleted of organic minerals and trace minerals and saturated with synthetic fertilizers and pesticides results in food that does not contain the raw material for our defense system to restock and rebuild itself.

In my experience, seldom do people die from a diagnosed disease. When people are very ill, they usually become dehydrated and experience sleep deprivation. Both conditions can further weaken the immune system, setting in motion a chain reaction of systemic failures that often hasten death.

Our Hippocrates wellness model for regenerating the immune system relies on a holistic, integrative approach. We use a combination of detoxification, the lifeforce of raw living food, specially selected whole food supplements, a balanced amount of rest and exercise, and generous doses of positive thinking to create a synergy that empowers the body to heal itself.

the role of nutrition

When we eat cooked food, our immune system reacts as if we have just been contaminated by an army of toxic invaders. Our white blood cells mobilize in large numbers and spring into action to annihilate this foreign army. The more cooked food we eat, the more our immune system is in a perpetual frenzy of activity. This depletes its energy and diminishes its effectiveness in maintaining health and fighting some of the more dangerous microbes and chemical toxins once they enter and colonize our system.

These findings about the immune-suppressing effects of cooked food, especially meat, came to light in 1930 at the First International Congress of Microbiology in Paris. Paul Kouchakoff, a Swiss physician, reported his discovery that eating cooked food produces leukocytosis—an elevation of white corpuscles in the blood—but the consumption of raw food does not produce these higher white cell counts.

While at the University of Clinical Chemistry in Switzerland, Dr. Kouchakoff performed three hundred experiments on the relationship between white cell counts and cooked versus raw food. He reached the conclusion that the effect was a pathological response of the human body to any food altered by high temperatures. Previously, medical science had considered this elevation to be a natural physiological phenomenon. He further observed that prepared or processed meat, when cooked or smoked, brought on the most violent reaction from the human immune system, which mobilized white blood cells in numbers comparable to when the body is poisoned by chemicals or pathogens.

An internal program review study that we conducted at Hippocrates from 1982 to 1983 confirmed these findings and drew a direct link between a raw vegan diet, immune system recovery, and the healing of catastrophic illnesses and diseases. We had 275 people participate in our study, and we measured their immune system effectiveness based on the percentages of cooked food they consumed.

We found that when cooked food comprises 25 to 30 percent of a person's diet (based on the overall weight of the food consumed), that individual's immunity is lowered by 17.6 percent. Any amount of cooked food beyond that percentage resulted in a 48 percent weakening of immune system cells. As a result of these findings, we advise anyone who is seriously ill to eat a totally raw vegan diet for two years to keep his or her immune system completely undistracted from the task of fighting the illness or disease.

We have observed that after people spend two years on a totally raw vegan diet, their immune system recovers and wellness follows. This is our natural lifeforce in action, doing the job that nature intended for it.

Support for our observations about the positive results of raw food on immunity has come from numerous medical science studies. A 1990 study from Germany, for instance, described how raw food positively influences the health of the immune system. These effects include antibiotic, antiallergic, anti-inflammatory, and tumor-protective actions.

At the Oregon Health and Science University, researchers monitored the immune systems of forty-two adult monkeys for forty-two months. Half were fed a nutritious, reduced-calorie diet; the other half got a traditional monkey diet. Monkeys on the nutritious, reduced-calorie diet had much better T-cell function. This study appeared in a December 2006 issue of the *Proceedings of the National Academies of Science*.

More than seventy studies on humans have found that beta-carotene, which is abundant in green, germinating seeds such as alfalfa and sunflower greens, can act as an antioxidant to neutralize the free radicals that damage cells and contribute to cancer. This nutrient directly enhances the immune system in a way that protects against tumors, particularly lung cancer and melanoma.

the many roles of wheatgrass

Wheatgrass juice contains one of nature's highest concentrations of chlorophyll, which is a key component of lifeforce energy. A series of laboratory experiments and reports over seven decades have identified chlorophyll as a therapeutic tonic for a wide range of illnesses and diseases. Here are a few of these findings:

- An article in *Journal of Biological Chemistry* extolled chlorophyll as therapeutic in the treatment of anemia, tuberculosis, arteriosclerosis, and other disorders. Another study appearing in that same science journal and a second study in *American Journal of Surgery* documented the effectiveness of chlorophyll as a tissue growth stimulator and a healing agent for numerous types of ulcers.

- A study appearing in *Gastroenterology* found chlorophyll effective with both ulcers and colon disorders. In that experiment, seventy-nine patients with gastric ulcers were treated with chlorophyll and fifty-eight showed complete healing within two to seven weeks of starting its use. There was no recurrence of symptoms in any of these patients.

- It was established that chlorophyll inhibits the putrefaction of protein by bacteria commonly found in the colons of meat eaters.
- At least four studies done in the 1950s showed that chlorophyll-rich foods (such as kale) enabled research animals to survive while undergoing high-radiation treatments.

the role of nutriceuticals

Nutritional supplements have a role to play in keeping our immune systems healthy, but at least 90 percent of the nutriceuticals being sold today, rather than being directly extracted from plant sources, are fabricated by pharmaceutical companies, which mix petrochemicals with other synthetic chemicals.

We recommend only using nutriceuticals that are whole food supplements, directly produced from food, herbs, enzymes, and their derivatives. These contain all of the cofactor constituents, the combination of nutrients that produce a positive synergistic effect that synthetic chemicals cannot duplicate.

During a two-year internal program review study at Hippocrates, we tested the value of nutriceuticals in immune system functioning and healing. We separated 284 people into two groups based upon the relative strength or weakness of the cells in their immune systems. Blood tests determined each person's physiology based on the numbers of white blood cells (leukocytes), T cells, H cells, and a range of differentials. The study participants were of both genders and represented a wide range of ages, occupations, levels of physical activity, and ethnic origins.

Those who displayed moderate immune strength were placed into the "healthy" group, which also included people who evidenced abundant immune strength and excellent health. In the "unhealthy" group were those with moderately weak blood test results and those displaying minimal immune function. Each participant followed an individually prescribed nutriceutical program.

Our 1994 study revealed that taking the immune-building supplements resulted in a 26 percent average increase in immune system efficiency among the "unhealthy" group. This degree of nutritional fulfillment can frequently be the difference between life and death.

regenerating an entire immune system

In 1998, I dislocated vertebrae in my spinal cord after lifting a heavy box at work. Within months of the trauma, I was diagnosed with fibromyalgia and chronic fatigue syndrome, and I went on disability leave from my work as a certified public accountant and auditor for an international accounting firm. Within a year after the injury, my immune system crashed completely.

I constantly battled infections and colds. Yeast rampaged throughout my body. Pain and insomnia were constant companions. My digestive tract shut down. I became bloated and gained ninety pounds in just one year. My immunologist diagnosed me with a T-cell defect in my immune system and explained that I was living like someone with advanced AIDS but without the virus.

I went on gamma globulin treatments, but they did little to boost my immune system function. Each year I would experience more and more health challenges: irritable bowel syndrome, fatty lipomas, high cholesterol, hypoglycemia, hormonal imbalance, chronic sinus infections, and chemical sensitivities.

In the summer of 2004, an alternative doctor put me on a diet of live foods that alkalize the body, and a radical shift began to take place. For the first few months, as my body detoxified, I felt much worse, with increased fatigue. But within three or four months of alkalizing my body, I began to show marked improvement. My blood pressure normalized, and one by one, my symptoms began to disappear.

After about six months, I was able to walk without the use of a cane. In May of 2006, I attended the three-week Hippocrates Program. My health continued to improve. I actually began strength training and cardiovascular exercise. As the months have gone by, I have continued to strengthen my body through raw food and exercise. My husband, Pierre, and I now wholeheartedly enjoy this new life that we have together.

DENISE SASIAIN, MIAMI
FLORIDA

Within the "healthy" group, immune-enhancing progress was also found, but it averaged a more modest 7 percent. While this percentage may seem minimal, it is nonetheless critical for people who expend great amounts of energy in their daily lives, such as athletes, pregnant women, and people who travel often.

Both groups reported increased stamina, strength, clarity, and overall physical functioning. The study also determined that most of the participants in both groups needed to consume nutriceutical supplements for about two years in order to regenerate the balance of their immune cells and achieve complete immune system functioning. Most of the participants continue to take these compact power-nutrients in an effort to stave off premature aging and disease.

One of the most potent nutriceuticals is green and blue-green algae, single-cell life-forms that are chlorophyll rich and promote cell building and immune fortification. A team of medical researchers at Royal Victoria Hospital in Canada examined how the brand-name product Super Blue-Green Algae strengthens the human immune system. As they reported in 1998, their double-blind study of fifty people found that after eating 1.5 grams of this algae, NK (natural killer) cell activity within the immune system increased significantly for the study participants. These immune cells were stimulated by the algae to move from the bloodstream into body tissues to scavenge for sick cells and toxic invaders. Other studies of this immune system booster have found it effective in reducing cholesterol.

Blue-green algae was the first life-form on the planet that created oxygen to spawn all other life-forms that would emerge. It truly is primal nutrition that benefits the human body at the cellular and DNA levels. We now routinely give it to all of our guests in supplement and liquid form. These extraordinary foods feed the brain like nothing else and help to rebuild its structure and prevent attention deficit disorder (ADD) and memory loss.

The following is a list and brief discussion of those whole food nutriceuticals that are most often utilized to enhance health and healing:

green and blue-green algae. A staple of the Hippocrates Program, these chlorophyll-rich, single-cell life-forms supply complete proteins and help maintain and strengthen red blood cells and the organs they support. They also promote cell building and fortify DNA.

flower pollens. Often used to relieve airborne allergies, flower pollens also provide vitamins, minerals, and complete proteins that facilitate building muscle, brain cells, and tissue.

food-grown supplements and cultured whole food supplements. Extracted from whole food or cultured food, nutrient-specific supplements contain the cofactors that facilitate absorption, thus increasing their effectiveness.

liquid ionic minerals. Most commercial mineral supplements cannot be easily digested, and rather than fulfilling the mineral needs of the body, they dilute minerals to alarmingly deficient levels. This is commonly caused by supplements that have a large molecular structure. The minute structure of ionic minerals makes these vital nutrients easy to digest and assimilate. A lack of minerals causes symptoms more quickly than any other nutritional deficiency.

sea vegetable supplements. Sea vegetables are rich in protein and chlorophyll and have exceptional amounts of most minerals and trace minerals. They help build healthy cells and promote glandular development.

the role of sleep and rest

onsistently restful sleep is one of the most overlooked yet crucial ways in which our bodies regenerate our immune system. Sleep restores, renews, and protects each cell in this wondrous community of cells.

Have you ever noticed, when you have a serious cold or the flu, how going to bed and getting a lot of sleep helps to rejuvenate your body so it recovers more quickly? By the same token, if you have a serious illness and are unable to sleep for more than a few hours at a time, recovery seems much slower and the resulting fatigue feels more debilitating.

A sleep-deprivation study conducted at the University of Chicago, published in the *Journal of the American Medical Association,* employed male and female athlete volunteers in their early twenties. They were permitted to sleep only four hours per night during a seven-day period. After a mere twenty-eight hours of lost normal sleep, they began manifesting the levels of mental and physical functioning typically seen in the average seventy-five-year-old. All of the bodily systems, especially immunity, degenerated.

Over a six-year period, a study by the American Cancer Society evaluated the health-promoting and health-damaging habits of one million people. This extensive study revealed that the highest mortality

immune system breakdown reversed

In 1998, at the age of forty-two, I was diagnosed with the beginning stages of multiple myeloma, a cancer of the plasma cells. Plasma cells are a vital part of the immune system, since they produce antibodies to fight infections. Therefore, anyone with multiple myeloma has a compromised immune system.

Previously a disease that affected only elderly people, multiple myeloma is increasingly being diagnosed in younger adults. Researchers speculate that it is caused by a combination of genetics and exposure to heavy metals, pesticides, and other chemical toxins. There is no known medical cure.

Naturally, I had no idea what multiple myeloma was when I received the diagnosis. My doctor advised that we continue tracking my condition and that eventually I would need to undergo chemotherapy and have a bone marrow transplant. My first question to her was, "In the meantime, what should I eat? What can I do?" She advised me to continue my normal diet. Rather than wait passively for my condition to worsen, I decided to research alternatives. I took my fate into my own hands.

One day, while I was at the health food store, a lady backed into my car in the parking lot. The first thing she said to me was that she was sure we met for a reason. When she gave me her business card, it turned out that she worked at the Hippocrates Health Institute. That was my introduction to the Hippocrates Program. Shortly thereafter, I enrolled in the program and embraced it fully.

In 2002, at the insistence of my hematologist, I had a bone marrow biopsy. She was sure it was time for me to have a bone marrow transplant. The results of the biopsy read as follows: "Marrow aspirate showing no immunophenotypic evidence of residual multiple myeloma." In lay terms that means no cancer! It has been seven years now, and I am more alive and healthier than ever.

JUANITA GONZALES
WEST PALM BEACH, FLORIDA

rates—for all age groups—occurred among those who slept four hours or less per night and those who slept nine or more hours per night. The lowest mortality rate was among those who got eight hours of uninterrupted sleep per night.

We at Hippocrates consider sleep—in conjunction with a positive attitude, the consumption of raw living food, and consistent exercise—to be essential lifeforce ingredients for health. Our research has led us to modify our position regarding the use of sleep aids. If you have diligently pursued some form of meditation, prayer, contemplation, or other relaxation techniques, and have still been unable to sleep restfully, we recommend trying some of the Asian herbal formulas that are on the market. If those fail, then as a last resort we recommend the temporary use of prescription medicines, which, despite their potential side effects, are preferable to the devastating effects on immunity of long-term sleep loss.

The ideal pattern of sleep is to retire shortly after sundown and arise shortly after sunrise. A brief midday nap—the siesta—can be beneficial in further recharging the immune system. The lengthy list of celebrated afternoon nappers includes Thomas Edison, Buckminster Fuller, Mahatma Gandhi, and Albert Einstein. Unfortunately, given our high-speed lifestyles and work routines, many people can aspire to these respites only on weekends or special occasions.

the role of exercise

With good nutrition and whole foods, you are well on the way to enhancing your immunity. But there is another important piece to the puzzle of boosting the immune system—exercise. Fascinating research from Loma Linda University in California demonstrates that even moderate exercise strengthens the immune system and reduces the likelihood of illness.

Fifty women who did not normally exercise were put into two groups—one group took a brisk, forty-five-minute walk for five days a week, while the other group remained sedentary. During the fifteen-week trial, the sedentary group was sick an average of ten days, whereas the walkers were sick for only five days. Natural killer and other immune cells increased in the women who walked but not in the sedentary group.

One theory about how exercise boosts immunity is that exercise releases antibodies, which attach themselves to viruses or bacteria and destroy them, according to David Nieman, chairman of the Health Science Department at Loma Linda. He says, "Walking seems to prime the immune system so that it's ready for action."

regenerated immune system does the real healing

My hell began with the words, "You have an inoperable cancer, and it's your leg or your life!" My orthopedic oncologist spoke those words after failing in an attempt to surgically remove the tumor in my left knee. "I can't guarantee your survival after the amputation," he continued, "but it's a start."

Shortly thereafter, the medical team advised my husband, C. S., to contact hospice; clearly the prognosis was not optimistic. We were devastated. I could not believe that I could be losing my leg or my life or both. I decided to submit to an experimental hyperthermic isolated limb perfusion—a drastic, localized, chemo-therapeutic procedure. The procedure itself was grueling, but the worst part was that the operating oncologist removed—without forewarning me—all of the lymph nodes in my left groin area. I had lost an essential part of my immune system for no reason, because the lymph nodes had tested negative for cancer.

My health challenges continued. I contracted a severe, life-threatening infection due to a poorly attached drain in my leg. I was rehospitalized. My condition worsened, and I believed that I was nearing death. I decided to forgo all of my medications, thinking that these might be causing more harm than good. Meanwhile, we were racing the clock to find a place where I could recover, free from further poisoning.

During more vigorous exercise, the brain releases endorphins, chemicals that give the feeling of a natural high. Some evidence has emerged that endorphins energize certain types of immune system cells. Because aerobic workouts raise body temperature, it is also possible that the heat helps to eliminate some viruses and bacteria.

A 2006 study published in *Cell Biochemistry and Function* presented evidence that moderate physical activity performed on a regular basis strengthens the immune system to resist both infections and cancer growth, in large part because the numbers of immune cells grow, causing them to circulate more quickly. "The entire mechanism by which exer-

We found the Hippocrates Program, and both my husband and I checked in and made all of the recommended lifestyle changes. We continued with the program after leaving Hippocrates. Within a year, a follow-up MRI revealed that the sarcoma behind my knee had diminished from 42 to 27 millimeters in diameter, and it had completely disentangled from the neurovascular bundle of blood vessels, nerves, and connecting tissues. The doctor handed the MRI to my husband, turned toward me, and said one word, "Congratulations!" Of course, we were moved to tears. This time, though, they were tears of joy.

My last MRI was in November 2001. The tumor had reduced in volume by over 90 percent and was well on its way to being eradicated by my dramatically improved immune system. The radiologist, comparing this MRI to the original one from 1996, said with amazement that in his twenty-five years in radiology he had never seen this type of reversal. The head oncologist was equally amazed. He was not only baffled that I had full use of my leg again, but also that the tumor had retracted and was nearly gone. I asked him if he would like to know what I had done to get these amazing results. To my amazement, he replied, "I don't have time to learn about that."

Today, even without those lymph nodes, my wonderful immune system has cleared away almost all of the damage and constructed new, healthy tissues. My leg looks great and feels almost the same as my other leg. I am bursting with energy and have vibrant health. And my husband and I have become accomplished ballroom dancers.

ALICE STERN
WEST PALM BEACH, FLORIDA

cise makes the immune system aware of challenges remains mostly uncovered," said the team of researchers who authored this study. However, research shows that active muscle cells produce more glutamine (an amino acid), and exercise more than doubles the number of macrophage cells (cells that destroy foreign antigens) circulating in the bloodstream.

While moderate exercise is an immune booster, there is a tipping point that can cause an overly strenuous workout to have the opposite effect. Maximum exertion for long periods of time temporarily exhausts the immune response. When the Loma Linda research team observed what happened to athletes who competed in the Los Angeles

Marathon, they found that the extreme exertion weakened the runners' immune systems for several hours afterward. There seems to be a window of three to twelve hours after heavy-endurance exercise in which the immune system is weak and vulnerable, apparently the result of the stress hormones cortisol and adrenaline having been released.

Impaired immune function has been associated with poor nutrition, fatigue, lack of sleep, stress, and poor lifestyle habits. It has long been known and observed in medical circles that stress, especially in the aftermath of a spouse's death or other types of psychological trauma, depresses the immune system to the point that illness, disease, and even death can soon follow.

the roles of imagination and emotion

Some years ago, one of our guests at Hippocrates walked into my office carrying a four-inch pile of medical reports from three physicians. After I had read this mass of material thoroughly, he asked my opinion about his cancer, which had metastasized throughout his body, from his vital organs to his skeletal structure. When I replied that it was diagnostically impossible for all three oncologists to be wrong, he whisked the papers out of my hands, called me a few choice names, and slammed the door on his way out.

About a year later he showed up again at my office with another barrage of verbal assaults, the gist of which was that all the doctors, and I, had been stunningly wrong about his condition. I started to defend myself when I suddenly realized that his belief had been more powerful than absolute physical reality. Years later, when he was well into his eighties, this man continued to flourish in good health and with a positive attitude.

Western medical science used to be steadfast in its insistence that the human immune system worked independently of other systems of the body. This was based on the fact that if we place a T cell in a test tube, it will continue to battle toxins for a period of time. Thus, thoughts and feelings were treated as being disconnected from bodily responses.

That model of immunity changed when a large body of research emerged in the field of psychoneuroimmunology showing the numerous ways in which our emotions and beliefs influence our physical well-being. Thoughts and feelings generate chemical and electrical changes in the body that influence the functioning of the immune system. This process begins within the limbic system of the brain. From there, emotional information flows to receptor sites found in our endocrine glands, traveling via those complex chains of amino acids called neuropeptides.

Monocytes, key components of the immune system, have receptor sites for these same neuropeptides. Research has found that nerve tissue running through every major organ of the body links the immune system to the central nervous system through these monocytes. When we suppress emotions, the encoded neuropeptides continually search for receptor sites, without success. It is like a computer program glitch that causes a dysfunctional repetition of patterns.

Cell biologist Bruce Lipton, whose work is described in Chapter 2, has spent much of his career investigating how positive thinking directly empowers the cells of our immune system to fight disease and regenerate the body. "The brain controls the behavior of the body's cells," he writes in *The Biology of Belief.* "The fact is that harnessing the power of your mind can be more effective than the drugs you have been programmed to believe you need."

Single cells within our body possess a level of intelligence, says Lipton, who has demonstrated this effect in laboratory experiments. "When cells band together in creating multicellular communities, they follow the 'collective voice' of the organism, even if that voice dictates self-destructive behavior." That collective voice in humans is a synchronous harmony between the conscious mind and the subconscious mind in setting an intention for healing.

Body/mind researchers have documented direct links between stress—which suppresses immune activity—and the development of cancer and heart disease. Emotional stress creates hormone imbalances and stimulates the production of abnormal cells. Our immune system normally sweeps away cancer cells as if they were dust or dirt, but like a housecleaner who becomes fatigued from stress and overwhelmed by the resulting accumulation of dust, our immune cells can become stressed and overworked until they stop cleaning properly.

Studies conducted at the Institute of HeartMath, a California research center devoted to the study of heart physiology and emotions, detail how stressful feelings can increase our risk of developing heart disease. Negative emotions set up a chain reaction within the body that causes stress hormone levels to increase, blood vessels to constrict, blood pressure to rise, and the immune system to become fatigued. Sustained stress burdens the heart by causing erratic heart rhythms.

twelve immune system boosters

1. Get outdoors and into the sun. For twenty to thirty minutes daily, get direct and/or indirect sunlight. The best times are before 9:00 a.m. and after 3:00 p.m. in the winter, or after 6:00 p.m. in the summer. Allow the full-spectrum sunlight to enter your eyes by not wearing sunglasses during this time. The sun is the most powerful immune system builder.

2. Consume adequate oxygen. Put yourself in or near oxygen-rich environments—oceans, forests, running streams, greenhouses—and learn to breathe deeply. Eat plenty of oxygen-rich green foods. If you are indoors for most of the day, purchase an oxygen-producing air purifier.

3. Drink pure water. The best water purification processes are distilled or molecule organized. Consume in ounces the amount equal to one-half your weight in pounds. Add safe, oxygen-enhancing products to your drinking water.

4. Eat a totally vegan diet that is comprised of 75 percent or more raw food by volume. Sprouts and green vegetables are the most balanced and nourishing choices.

5. Drink freshly made beverages from sprouted green vegetables twice a day.

Conversely, research from the Institute of HeartMath shows that when we experience the positive emotions of love, compassion, and appreciation, our heart produces a smooth, rhythmic pattern, which enhances cardiovascular efficiency. If we can summon a past memory that evokes warm emotional feelings, we strengthen our heart and immune system. "It's important to emphasize," says Rollin McCraty, director of research at HeartMath, "that it is not a mental image of a memory that creates a shift in our heart rhythm, but rather the emotions associated with the memory. We have seen significant results when someone focuses on a positive feeling."

Lab work done by Candace B. Pert, author of *Molecules of Emotion: The Science Behind Mind-Body Medicine*, has demonstrated that

6. Use "regular" blue-green algae. Super blue-green algae or Hawaiian spirulina, along with chlorella, are high-quality concentrated foods that enhance immunity.

7. Stop using immune-suppressing ingredients. These include salt, refined sugars and flours, dairy products, vinegars, heated oils, and food preservatives, additives, stabilizers, and colorings.

8. Avoid microwaved and fried foods, which can suppress the immune system and lead to cancers and heart and circulatory diseases.

9. Eliminate alcohol and drugs. Unless your prescriptions are absolutely essential to your survival, stop taking them. Alcohol and drugs do not mix, except to undermine our immune systems.

10. Exercise moderately. Engage in stretching, aerobic, and resistance exercises at least five times a week for thirty to sixty minutes a day.

11. Get adequate rest. Sleep and rest helps to recharge the immune system. As part of this strategy, rest the entire body once a week on a juice-and-water fast. This enables the immune system to do a weekly cleanup.

12. Keep a smile on your face. Maintaining a positive attitude is key to having a belief system that supports immunity. Read the book *Anatomy of an Illness* by Norman Cousins for a primer on how laughter and humor can enhance the human immune system. Nature, color, sound, music, and laughter can positively affect the immune system.

peptide molecules in the body stimulated by strong emotions can direct the traffic of tumor cells. Her data shows that tumor progression, or regression, is affected by people's attitudes about life.

Two pioneers in putting this body/mind connection into practice were oncologist O. Carl Simonton and psychologist Stephanie Simonton, who developed a visualization program for cancer patients after Carl Simonton observed that the people who experienced spontaneous remission from cancer were often those who declared, "I always imagined myself as well." The Simontons coached 159 cancer patients, who had been given less than a year to live, on using a visualization technique that consisted of seeing the white blood cells of their immune system swarm over the cancerous cells and destroy them.

Some people were able to master this concentration on visual images, while others were not so committed or successful. Yet, after two years, nearly half of the cancer "incurables" were still alive, and 22 percent of them no longer showed any signs of cancer in their bodies.

life-altering disorders in remission

When I was eight years old, my spleen ruptured and doctors had to remove it. During the procedure, they removed a part of my intestines. Subsequently, and throughout my childhood, I was sick every year with colds and flu infections that lasted for weeks. In addition, I began to lose the hearing in my left ear.

My health challenges continued into adulthood, and I began contracting systemic infections. Shortly after I was married, I developed spinal meningitis and nearly died. My body was covered with sores. I had hypertension, high cholesterol, and an arthritic disk in my back. I had constant pain in my neck and arms.

In March 2003, I had a massive grand mal seizure. During a CAT scan, it was discovered that I had a lesion—a large tumor—in my brain, in an area that was considered inoperable. The tumor had been growing for so long that it had become interwoven into the brain tissue. My doctor stated that it would have to grow until 70 percent of it could be surgically removed. If I survived this procedure, I would need to undergo radiation and chemotherapy.

I was no longer able to work or play with my children, and I was sleeping eighteen to twenty hours a day. During this period, a friend told me about the Hippocrates Program and said that it had helped both him and his mother. So my parents sent me to experience the Institute's program. Though it was difficult, I persevered and have remained loyal to the diet and lifestyle. This began an incredible transformation in me. All of my life-altering disorders—the high blood pressure, excess cholesterol, chronic pain, and even the activity of my tumor—have either disappeared or gone into remission. According to my latest MRI, there are two dead spots in the middle of the tumor and the swelling is gone. I am now the healthiest that I have ever been.

BRIAN TOUW, BLOOMINGDALE
NEW JERSEY

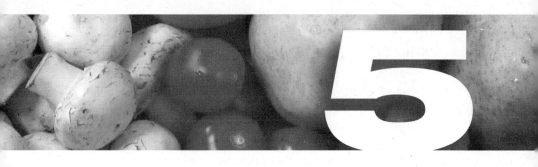

how our food becomes medicine

Our food should be our medicine.
Our medicine should be our food.

HIPPOCRATES

W hen the Greek physician Hippocrates stated more than 2,300 years ago that food is medicine, he spoke from a knowledge that had been gained by astute observation and sharp intuition. He observed the many positive effects that food could have on human health, and he intuited that people possessed what we now know to be an immune system, a healing potential within the body, a potent lifeforce that could be harnessed using food as fuel.

Recent human advances in understanding nutrition and its effect on human immunity have provided us with a wealth of unassailable research data showing that the wisdom of Hippocrates transcends time. Britain's Institute of Food Research, for instance, in a 2002 review of all nutrigenomics research up until that date (nutrigenomics is a new field of study concerned with the ways in which food consumption can affect whether our genes will trigger disease), came to this firm conclusion: "Evidence that diet is a key environmental factor affecting the incidence of many chronic diseases is overwhelming. The food we eat contains thousands of biologically active substances, many of which may have the potential to provide substantial health benefits."

As should now be clear to all fair-minded people, our diets can prevent disease, cause disease, or provide the lifeforce energy to heal illness and disease. Central to determining the path our bodies will take is the quality and quantity of the nutrients we absorb. Seven nutrients are known to be essential to sustain the human body. Without a constant infusion of these nutrients from natural food, your body and mind would deteriorate.

Another entire family of nutrients essential to health and healing are phytochemicals, also known as phytonutrients. Only within the past few decades has the discovery been made that these compounds, which are

TABLE 3: *the seven essential nutrients*

NUTRIENT	SOURCES AND/OR PURPOSE
Lipids	Lipids include essential fatty acids that help to build and maintain all of the body's organs, including the brain.
Minerals and trace minerals	Minerals and trace minerals provide the physical foundation and circuitry for the electrical conductivity of the entire body/mind.
Oxygen	Oxygen is the most important element of all. We get it from the air we breathe and from the foods we eat.
Probiotics	Probiotics are bacteria that are beneficial for us because they support all bodily functions from digestion to elimination, as well as the development and maintenance of the immune system. For more information on probiotics, see Chapter 12.
Proteins	Proteins which are made up of amino acids, have both structural and functional roles in the body. Though some amino acids are naturally part of our system, many others must be derived from food or its nutriceutical extracts.
Vitamins	Vitamins are unique nutrients found in food that require frequent restocking within our bodies.
Water	Without water all life would perish. We get water directly from drinking it and indirectly from the food we eat.

produced naturally by plants as a protection against pests and diseases, play such an important role in our own well-being. Phytochemicals contain protective, disease-preventing compounds that interact with other plant nutrients to produce a synergy that can help prevent or treat cancer, diabetes, cardiovascular disease, and hypertension.

The online encyclopedia *Wikipedia* describes the health benefits of phytonutrients this way: "What is beyond dispute is that phytonutrients have many and various salubrious functions in the body. For example, they may promote the function of the immune system, act directly against bacteria and viruses, reduce inflammation, and be associated with the treatment and/or prevention of cancer, cardiovascular disease, and any other malady affecting the health or well-being of an individual."

Phytochemicals even protect cartilage in the joints of our body and prevent joint pain and other symptoms of arthritis. Johns Hopkins University researchers published a study in a 2005 issue of the *Proceedings of the National Academy of Sciences* pointing out how these plant-derived compounds block the activity of an enzyme that triggers inflammation in joints. A Johns Hopkins School of Medicine press release described even more research findings about phytochemicals by the same medical team: "They detoxify certain cancer-causing agents and damaging free radicals in tissue, including cells that line blood vessels. These phytochemicals can be found in cruciferous plants, including broccoli."

More than one thousand different phytochemicals have been identified in plants, including flavonoids in fruits and lycopene in tomatoes. When herbicides and pesticides are used in nonorganic farming, plants do not produce nearly as many phytochemicals as they would under normal conditions. Time of harvest is another important consideration in the concentration of phytochemicals in food. Individual nutrients, phytochemicals, and enzymes reach optimal concentrations at distinct stages of plant growth. Early harvesting limits the health benefits derived from the consumption of these foods. Combined with the negative effects of food processing and cooking, both of which eliminate still more phytochemicals, it's no wonder the produce that most people consume today contains few health-protective benefits.

A good illustration of the dramatic differences in the health-supporting benefits between organic and nonorganic vegetables comes from a medical study done in Europe. Organic vegetables contain almost six times as much salicylic acid as nonorganic vegetables, according to a 2002 study in the *European Journal of Nutrition*. This helps to explain why eating organic food can reduce our risk of heart attacks, strokes, and cancer, because salicylic acid acts as an anti-inflammatory to combat both bowel cancer and hardening of the arteries. This study attributed the higher salicylic acid levels in organic vegetables to their natural production of the chemical as a defense against stress and disease, a process that is disrupted by the pesticides used in nonorganic farming.

Food manufacturers and the chemical and pharmaceutical industries are trying to capitalize on this new research about the health benefits of phytochemicals by creating synthetic versions in laboratories and marketing them as supplements or adding them to processed foods and proclaiming their health benefits. These "phony phytos" do not in any way resemble the natural compounds produced by nature. The necessary synergistic interactions that produce healing results are simply not present in synthetics.

"Nutrition represents the combined activities of countless food substances. The whole is greater than the sum of its parts," writes T. Colin Campbell in *The China Study*. "The chemicals we get from the foods we eat are engaged in a series of reactions that work in concert to produce good health. Everything in food works together to create health or disease. The more we think that a single chemical characterizes a whole food, the more we stray into idiocy." For more information on phytochemicals, see Chapter 12.

nature heals
what synthetics cannot

Every prescription drug carries several high prices—the cost of purchasing it and the costs exacted on health from the side effects of using it. Consider the three most common drugs prescribed for type 2 diabetes, which afflicts more than 200 million people worldwide. The *New England Journal of Medicine* reported in December 2006 how a study of diabetes patients using Avandia, the newest drug for this illness, found it was not only more expensive than the older drugs metformin and glyburide, it also raised the user's risk of heart problems, excessive weight gain, and bone fractures. The two older drugs generate serious side effects too, conceded the study authors, so it was really a case of choose your poison.

Compare these costly and risky drugs to what medical studies have found when a person uses a diet of natural vegan foods instead of drugs to treat diabetes. Nature's food chemicals are cheaper, more effective, and possess no side effects other than the benefit of improved overall health.

In the August 2006 issue of the medical journal *Diabetes Care*, the results of a twenty-two-week study, funded by the National Institutes of Health, described the effects of a low-fat vegan diet on diabetes. This randomized, controlled trial used ninety-nine people with type 2 diabetes, half of whom were assigned to follow a strict, low-fat vegan diet. The other half were placed on a calorie- and portion-controlled diet that included some meat and dairy products. Those people on the vegan diet experienced significantly greater reductions in blood sugar levels, cholesterol, and body weight.

"The [vegan] diet appears remarkably effective, and all the side effects are good ones—especially weight loss and lower cholesterol," observed Neal Barnard, an associate professor of medicine at George Washington University and coauthor of the study. "I hope this study will rekindle interest in using diet changes first, rather than prescription drugs, to treat type 2 diabetes." A previous study coauthored by Dr. Barnard and published in a 2005 issue of the *American Journal of Medicine* discovered that a vegan diet increased insulin sensitivity and reduced body weight in overweight women who were not yet diabetic, which demonstrated that the diet could be effective in forestalling the onset of diabetes in people with risk factors for the disease.

Cancer is another illness that, along with diabetes, continues to wreak a widening swath of havoc on people's health worldwide, yet a tremendous amount of medical research has accumulated over the past half century showing that a plant-based diet can prevent and even reverse this disease. Conversely, this research also demonstrates that diets rich in animal and dairy products are among the chief causes of many types of cancer.

Here is how the Institute of Food Research, Britain's leading non-profit organization for research on food and health, frames these findings about the role of diet in cancer causation and prevention: "Diet appears to influence the incidence or risk of cancer in a variety of ways. For example, a diet rich in red meat has been linked to a higher incidence of bowel cancer, while the consumption of excessive alcohol and cured and smoked meat and fish products are apparently associated with cancer of the mouth and digestive system. By contrast, other foods, such as fruits and vegetables, appear to reduce the incidence of certain types of cancers. For example, there is convincing evidence that a diet rich in green leafy vegetables protects against lung and stomach cancers, and probably also against cancer of the mouth and pharynx. Other vegetables, such as broccoli, cauliflower, and brussels sprouts, appear to protect against bowel and thyroid cancer, while *Allium* vegetables (such as garlic and onions), citrus fruits, and tomatoes probably protect against lung, stomach, and bladder cancers."

On its Web site, the Institute writes: "There are different biochemical explanations for the relationships between different food groups and cancer. Foods that appear to increase risk, such as cured foods and alcohol, often contain specific chemicals known to cause cancer (carcinogens). By contrast, fruits and vegetables contain a range of 'bioactive' compounds, some of which are thought to act as natural pesticides within the plant. These compounds include those that reduce the toxicity of carcinogens. Other compounds include antioxidants, which help to prevent the harmful side effects of free radicals produced as a consequence of normal processes but which can damage cells and DNA in the body. This damage may lead to the uncontrollable cell division typical of cancer. At present, the daily requirement for the levels of these bioactive compounds is not known. However, it is likely that a diet rich in a variety of foods of plant-based origin will ensure an adequate selection of these beneficial compounds."

Research evidence for the link between plant-based nutrition and good health is so overwhelming, there really should be no debate anymore. What passes for debate is quite often merely a smoke screen generated by vested economic interests (such as the meat, dairy, and processed food industries) trying to protect their profits, or at the individual level it is a denial and rationalization designed to protect harmful and addictive lifestyle choices.

For those people who still harbor doubts about the healing powers of plant-based diets, or the disease consequences of consuming meat and dairy products, here is a sampling of the independent scientific research supporting the Hippocrates approach to diet and health.

all cancers

Several medical researchers placed cancer-causing chemicals in two types of food—natural, unrefined, unprocessed food versus refined and processed food that was low in vitamins and minerals—to test whether lab animals would develop cancer faster on one of the diets. Within twenty-two weeks, according to the journal *Cancer Research*, none of the animals on the unrefined diet had contracted cancer, but 90 percent of animals on the processed diet had developed liver and mammary tumors.

Japanese scientists studied the antitumor effects of sea vegetables commonly eaten in Asia, which are frequently prescribed by practitioners of Traditional Chinese Medicine to treat cancer, and found that they significantly inhibited the growth of tumors in lab animals. "The tumors underwent complete regression in more than half of the mice treated," observed the scientists, writing in the *Japanese Journal of Experimental Medicine* in 1974.

Researchers at the Linus Pauling Institute at Oregon State University, writing in a 2006 issue of *Carcinogenesis*, described how the phytochemical called indole-3-carbinol, found in broccoli and other cruciferous vegetables, protected pregnant mice and their offspring from leukemia, lung cancer, and lymphomas. This phytochemical seems to induce enzymes to detoxify carcinogens and may even cause mutant cells to commit suicide before they can do harm to the human body.

In a review of hundreds of science studies that examined the relationship between cancer and the consumption of fruits and vegetables, researchers writing in the journal *Nutrition and Cancer* in 1992 identified 128 studies showing that plant-based foods offer a significant protective effect against cancer. Overall, the relative risk of cancer was at least twice as low for people who ate the most plant-based foods.

colon cancer

In the medical journal *Carcinogenesis*, a 2004 study documented how allyl isothiocyanate (AITC), a plant chemical, sabotages the uncontrolled cell division of colon cancer cells. AITC is found in mustard, cabbage, horseradish, brussels sprouts, kale, and wasabi. According to the study's authors, AITC appears to selectively target tumor cells, unlike chemotherapeutic drugs, which also harm healthy cells.

In a 1992 edition of the *Journal of Nutrition*, a team of researchers reported that an uncooked, extreme vegan diet causes a decrease in bacterial enzymes and certain toxic products that have been implicated in colon cancer risk. Researchers at the Fox Chase Cancer Center in Philadelphia examined thirty-seven medical studies involving ten thousand people in fifteen countries and discovered that persons who had a high plant-based diet lowered their risk of colorectal cancer by at least 40 percent.

breast cancer

Women who eat red meat when they are in their twenties, thirties, and forties greatly increase their risk of contracting breast cancer, according to a Harvard University study of ninety thousand women published in the *Archives of Internal Medicine* during 2006. Researchers speculated that substances produced by cooking meat, along with naturally occurring substances in the meat itself, may combine to disrupt female hormones and trigger the onset of breast cancer.

bladder cancer

Certain natural compounds found in broccoli and broccoli sprouts interfere with the growth of bladder cancer cells, according to study done in 2005 by a team of researchers at Ohio State University. Broccoli sprouts are even more effective in killing cancer cells than broccoli, kale, brussels sprouts, and the other cruciferous vegetables that contain isothiocyanate, a compound that been identified as being biologically protective.

lung cancer

Scientists at University College, London, told the journal *Cancer Research* in 2005 how they had discovered that a natural compound found in many legumes and nuts blocks a key enzyme involved in tumor growth. When this compound was tested on mice with ovarian and lung cancers, it was found to sabotage tumor growth. It was also noted to be nontoxic, unlike conventional chemotherapy drugs.

Research conducted on eighteen thousand men found that chemicals present in broccoli, cabbage, and other cruciferous vegetables offer strong protection against lung cancer. This finding was reported in a 2000 issue of the *Lancet*.

A study of men in Chicago, published in a 1992 issue of *American Journal of Epidemiology*, reported that those who ingested 500 milligrams or more of dietary cholesterol a day, mostly from eggs, had twice the risk of lung cancer as men who ate less than that amount of cholesterol.

pancreatic cancer

Eating at least five portions a day of certain vegetables cuts the risk of developing pancreatic cancer by at least 50 percent, reported a 2005 issue of the medical journal *Cancer, Epidemiology, Biomarkers & Prevention*. Raw vegetables were found to be more protective than cooked vegetables. Among the most highly cancer-protective foods were onions, garlic, carrots, and dark leafy vegetables. "Finding strong confirmation that simple life choices can provide significant protection from pancreatic cancer may be one of the most practical ways to reduce the incidence of this dreadful disease," said study coauthor Elizabeth Holly, an epidemiologist at the University of California at San Francisco.

A study of risk factors for the development of pancreatic cancer, published in 1993 in the journal *Cancer Causes and Control*, found that high consumption of meat was a chief cause of this form of cancer.

leukemia

Favorable and fast effects in reducing leukemia cells in bone marrow were observed in ten of thirteen children with leukemia who were placed on low-protein, plant-based diets, according to the *Lancet* in 1965.

heart disease

A 1958 study in the *Lancet* reported that a diet high in fresh vegetables caused a significant decrease in arteriosclerosis after just four weeks, while another British study a year later found that the higher the level of a person's vegetable consumption, the less severe the number and range of heart disorders. In 1960, the *Journal of Nutrition* published a study describing how vegetable protein acts to lower cholesterol.

Broccoli consumption was found to reduce the risk of coronary heart disease death in a large-scale study of postmenopausal women, as reported in the *American Journal of Epidemiology* in 1999.

In the *Journal of Nutrition*, a 2006 study reported that broccoli, green beans, peas, corn, and carrots thwart the progression of atherosclerosis (artery-clogging plaques). One group of mice was placed on a vegetable diet, the other on a nonvegetable diet, and after sixteen weeks the arteries of both groups were examined. The vegetable-fed mice had 38 percent less incidence of atherosclerosis.

escaping a death sentence from pancreatic cancer

Back in the late 1990s, I found myself suffering fatigue, nausea, and constantly interrupted sleep brought on by the excruciating pain in my stomach. My physician conducted some investigative blood work, and the results appeared to be completely normal, but an ultrasound test revealed a 10-centimeter mass on my pancreas.

The doctor explained that if I were older, she would believe that the tumor was benign; however, because I was young, she suspected it might be cancer. Just that word instilled so much fear in my heart. The doctor said that my options were surgery, chemotherapy, and radiation.

Adding to my massive fatigue, I now began suffering the effects of depression. All I could think about was the cancer. I was reluctant to make plans for the future. Three months away seemed like an eternity. Five years certainly seemed impossible. Should I continue to tend to my home? Would I be alive next week?

Thank goodness my five daughters came and nurtured me. They adjusted their schedules and stayed with me at the onset of this sad period of my life. They described my color as gray-green. On top of all of this, the doctors finally admitted that although chemotherapy and radiation treatments were suggested, they ultimately would not make any difference in my case, nor would they prolong my life. They told me, "I am sorry, Samantha, get your house in order."

These crushing words disheartened me and brought me to the realization I had been written off. My children and I continued to search the medical literature and found that a twelve-month survival rate would be the most I could hope for. After exploring all the medical options, we finally concluded that there were none. Fortunately, we had all practiced meditation for many years, so we were somewhat familiar with natural living and methods for healing. Slowly, I pulled myself together by improving my lifestyle, which gave me enough energy to search out a place of healing.

That is when I came upon the Hippocrates Health Institute. It was reassuring to find that they had fifty years of experience. There were innumerable examples of people who had beaten the odds and brought about their own recovery from catastrophic disease. Their belief paralleled mine—we must learn to trust our body and its ability to heal itself.

As I stepped onto the Institute's grounds and met the staff, I felt at home and completely encouraged for the first time since my diagnosis of death. I remember thinking about what a different experience it was there versus the medical model that I had suffered at home. I slowly adopted the program and was aghast when I looked through a microscope and viewed cancer cells thriving on cooked food. This wrenched me into fully practicing the living food diet. Slowly but surely, my pallor gave way to a more acceptable color, and as time passed, my normal skin tones prevailed.

In addition to the diet, I used far-infrared therapy to gently heat my body up to 115 degrees F and made sure to include lots of massage and reflexology. I continued my meditation and creative visualization and drank copious amounts of wheatgrass juice.

After two years, the tumors had shrunk to less than half their original size. Before I knew it, I was in remission. Now I knew the cancer could be beaten. What made me realize that I was completely well was my busy schedule, the many days I spent on the golf course or swimming, and all the fruitful time I enjoyed with my five fantastic daughters.

Coming back to life shook my core and helped to remove my fears. Realizing I was now a walking, talking example of my body's own intelligence gave me the vigor to share this experience with my family and friends. Now, almost seven years later, I realize that this lifestyle requires focus, daily commitment, and constant follow-through.

Taking total responsibility for my health has not only brought about my own survival over the last seven years, it has elevated me to the understanding that life begins with me. Each of us has the authority and responsibility to move forward and change anything we want to in our lives. Like me, you can squelch any limitation presented to you.

SAMANTHA YOUNG
TORONTO, CANADA

By contrast, a ten-year study published in a 1964 issue of the *Journal of the Royal College of General Practitioners* found that heated animal products are a primary contributor to all forms of heart disease.

rheumatoid arthritis

In the British *Journal of Rheumatology*, a study was reported in 1997 involving forty-three rheumatoid arthritis patients who were divided into two groups—one group ate their ordinary omnivorous diet, while the other ate a raw vegan diet. Stool samples were taken from the patients before the intervention and again one month into the experiment. It was found that the microbial flora of the patients on the vegan diet had changed significantly in a way that brought about improvements in the patients' conditions.

Another study, published in the journal *Toxicology* in 2000, researched the effects of an uncooked vegan diet on rheumatoid diseases. The study used a series of objective measures, including pain levels, and determined that patients' conditions improved as a result of the antioxidants and lactobacilli inherent in the vegan foods. To further test whether a raw vegan diet was superior to a cooked vegan diet in relieving fibromyalgia symptoms, a study published in the *Scandinavian Journal of Rheumatology* compared two groups of women patients—one group was placed on a completely raw vegetable diet, the other on a cooked vegan diet. Those on the raw vegetable diet experienced less pain, less stiffness, and better sleep than the group eating the cooked vegan food.

cooking destroys lifeforce and creates toxins

We have a motto at Hippocrates: "It's not the food in your life, it's the life in your food." Cooking destroys the medicinal value of food. The lifeforce in raw food comes from enzymes in the food's cells that have an electromagnetic frequency that is similar to the electromagnetic frequency of our own body cells. Like a couple whose eyes meet in a moment of attraction, the two electrically charged forces are normally attracted to each other and merge. But when food is processed or cooked, the electronic frequency is impaired, preventing the nutrients from being absorbed into our cells.

Phytonutrients heated to more than 118 degrees F lose their molecular structure and become lifeless microbodies without a health-protective function. Eating cooked food also triggers a pathogenic response in our bodies whereby white blood cells normally used for healing by our immune system are diverted to attack the food molecules that our bodies construe as foreign invaders.

On the Raw Food Life Web site (http://www.rawfoodlife.com), where many science studies are posted demonstrating the link between cooking and the creation of toxins, an overview called *Nutrition's Dr. Jekyll & Mr. Hyde* describes the dangers this way: "Everyone knows that cooking food reduces its nutrition. But did you ever stop and wonder happens to those lovely vitamins, minerals, fats, carbs, and proteins once they're cooked? Where do they go? Do they just disappear? Unfortunately, they do not. Like Dr. Jekyll, they are horribly transformed by chemical reactions into nasty killers like Mr. Hyde . . . only we call them Mr. Carcinogen, Mr. Mutagen, and that arch-villain of all time, Mr. Free Radical!"

When New York City's Board of Health voted unanimously in 2006 to ban the use of trans fats in restaurants, it was not only an acknowledgment of a vast nationwide food experiment that had failed; it was an action that unintentionally revealed the dangers inherent in all cooked animal products.

Trans fats in the form of partially hydrogenated oils were invented to be a more healthful alternative to saturated animal fats such as butter. These synthetics ended up in everything from processed foods to doughnuts to french fries, and most everything else fried or baked. But medical studies began accumulating a mountain of data decades ago showing that trans fats cause heart disease and a range of other serious ailments.

The debate in New York over whether these harmful substances should be banned brought to light an interesting admission from mainstream nutritionists and the medical establishment. Many types of meats and dairy products naturally contain the same trans fats that were being outlawed as a danger to human health. In fact, according to the U.S. Food and Drug Administration, at least 21 percent of the trans fats that an average adult consumes each year come directly from animal products.

Doctors and scientists supporting the ban were frequently quoted as saying that trans fats are dangerous in almost any amount, yet none of them bothered to mention that animal products are also a worthy

overcoming a brain tumor

My story begins in 2004. A CAT scan showed that I had a very large mass on the right side of my brain. I was diagnosed with a brain tumor! I could not believe it. To make matters worse, I needed immediate surgery.

We waited two days to see the neurosurgeon. The doctor wanted to take sections of my tumor for a biopsy. My husband, Stuart, told them there was no way he would allow this procedure. Next thing we knew, I was dismissed from St. Mary's Hospital.

By this time, I was having difficulty speaking and was suffering terrible headaches. I could barely walk and had blurry vision. I also could not write. All my motor skills were not functioning, and I lost the ability to maintain bladder control.

Faced with this dead end, my husband and I discussed alternatives. We needed something immediate and close, so we called the Hippocrates Health Institute and spoke to the director, Brian Clement. We all knew that I was going to need surgery as soon as we could find a doctor to do it. Dr. Clement urged me to change my eating habits immediately. This meant no more coffee with hazelnut cream, no sugar, no flour, very little fruit, no meat, no chicken, no fish. Only raw living food, lots of wheatgrass, green drinks, lots of sprouts, and water with lemon. I had to make a major change in the way that I ate in order to save myself.

Several months later, I had my surgery at the National Institutes of Health (NIH) in Bethesda, Maryland. It lasted seven hours, and I lost seven pints of blood. The size of my atypical meningioma brain tumor was close to four pounds (the size of a grapefruit). My recovery time was five days in the hospital plus two days as an outpatient.

When we got home from the hospital, the first thing we did was buy a juicer to make my wheatgrass and green drinks. I started buying sprouts and wheatgrass and even started growing my own.

Two months later, I started feeling tired and my head was hurting again, so I had an MRI with contrast. They found two small tumors in my brain. Then my husband and I flew up to the National Institutes of Health and had another MRI with contrast. The doctors found one small tumor.

Since I had an aggressive brain tumor, the doctors wanted to do immediate radiation on my brain for six weeks, once a day. I knew what the effects of radiation would bring—and I knew that I would have a malignant tumor five to twenty-five years later somewhere else in my body. Stuart and I agreed that we would take an alternative route. After my surgery, I was very consistent with the Hippocrates Program at first, but as time went on, I slowly started to slack off by not juicing every day. Also, I started to eat the wrong types of food more frequently.

We spoke to Dr. Clement again, and he recommended no fruits, no carrots, no dairy, and absolutely no sugar. He then asked me if I had an ironing board, and I said, "Yes, why?" He wanted me to put my head on the floor and raise my legs on the ironing board, leaning up on the couch twice a day for fifteen minutes so the blood would rush to my head and help with the healing process. Knowing that Dr. Clement knew his stuff, I was willing to do what he asked of me. I was afraid of what could happen if I did not stick to the plan. I also went to an acupuncturist for two months, used aggressive Chinese herbs, wore a magnetic headband, drank green drinks and wheatgrass juice, and ate lots of different kinds of sprouts several times a day as well as other types of raw living food.

In November 2005, the week before I was supposed to start radiation, I kept stalling; I did not feel the need for radiation. I called my neurosurgeon and asked him for one more MRI with contrast. I told him that if anything showed up, I would go through radiation without a word. I got my wish. I knew in my heart there would be nothing there. They did another MRI with contrast, and the findings showed no more tumors, no blood clots, no more hemorrhaging. All the doctors could say was that I did not need radiation. In May 2006, we went to the NIH for my three-month checkup. I had another MRI with contrast. The white-matter disease was gone. I had made it through.

BONNIE LOVETT
WEST PALM BEACH, FLORIDA

target for future legislative action. This glaring omission demonstrates not only the economic clout of the meat and dairy industries, but reveals how many of the so-called health experts are people so personally addicted to a meat-and-dairy diet that they are in denial about the dangers that are posed to even their own health.

Right in the midst of this debate over trans fats in New York, a study surfaced in Britain that raised equally disturbing questions about the health effects of using high temperatures to cook food. The *Journal of Agricultural and Food Chemistry* reported that flour from wheat grown in sulfur-deprived soils (which characterizes most of our mineral-depleted croplands) creates dangerously high levels of acrylamide, a carcinogen, when it is exposed to high heat during cooking. Foods such as potato chips, cookies, and bread contain the highest levels of acrylamide. Microwaving foods can also create it.

Acrylamide has been linked to male reproductive damage and neurological disorders, and it may also play a role in the development of many cancers. Harvard Medical School researchers observed in a 2005 issue of the *International Journal of Cancer* that girls who eat potato chips and french fries increase their chances of getting breast cancer when they become adults.

Hippocrates founder, Ann Wigmore, often talked about how the most thrilling experience she could recall was to see cancer cells taken from a human body thrive on cooked food, but these cells were unable to survive on the same food when it was uncooked.

Besides creating toxins that directly endanger human health, cooking also destroys most of the lifeforce in food, obliterating the many phytochemicals, vitamins, minerals, and enzymes essential to the maintenance of good health. Studies done over the past few years at the Linus Pauling Institute at Oregon State University found that boiling cruciferous vegetables such as broccoli for just nine minutes destroys 59 percent of the phytochemical indole-3-carbinol, which has been identified in other studies at this research facility as being a potent inhibitor of cancer cell growth.

Our bodies do not naturally produce vitamin B_{12}, which is important for the proliferation of red blood cells and the support of our nervous system; it is also vital for development during childhood. At Hippocrates, we did an internal program review in 2005 that tested one hundred of our guests for vitamin B_{12} and other vitamin and mineral deficiencies. We found that 80 percent had some type of mineral deficiency, while 60 percent lacked adequate levels of vitamin B_{12}. Since our bodies are essentially electrical systems, especially our hearts and brains, we need adequate levels of minerals in our diets to facilitate the movement of electrons throughout the body. Mineral deficiencies have been linked to both Parkinson's disease and multiple sclerosis.

The test we used involved intracellular blood analysis, which shows us which nutrients are actually absorbed by the cells. Unlike traditional blood testing, which can produce skewed results if supplements have been taken, the Functional Intracellular Analysis test provides a picture of how well the body's white blood cells are nourished by micronutrients. This relatively new technology, developed at the University of Texas, exposes antioxidant levels in the body, specific nutrient depletions, and lipid and protein levels as they relate to cardiovascular disease.

Enzymes in food are particularly sensitive to the high temperatures of cooking. These specialized proteins accelerate chemical reactions within our cells, which means they play a role equivalent to spark plugs within cellular engines, making them responsible for keeping the entire bodily system functioning properly. Digestive enzymes break down the food we consume, while thousands of other types of enzymes act as catalysts, each with a specialized role.

the health role of enzymes

Wikipedia describes the role of enzymes in disease processes this way: "The importance of enzymes is shown by the fact that a lethal illness can be caused by the malfunction of just one type of enzyme out of thousands of types present in our bodies."

Certain raw organic foods are natural stimulators of the detoxifying enzymes our bodies need to combat cancer and other diseases. Researchers from Johns Hopkins University School of Medicine discovered in 1997 that broccoli sprouts, as opposed to the more familiar broccoli heads, are powerful stimulators of natural detoxifying enzymes in the human body.

Here is how the *New York Times,* on September 16, 1997, described these benefits in an article announcing the discovery: "Broccoli sprouts contain anywhere from thirty to fifty times the concentration of protective chemicals found in mature broccoli plants.

These chemicals, called isothiocyanates, were already known to be potent stimulators of natural detoxifying enzymes in the body, and are thought to help explain why the consumption of broccoli and other cruciferous vegetables like cauliflower, cabbage, and kale is associated with a lowered risk of contracting cancer."

This article quoted scientists involved in the research as extolling the enzyme-enhancing virtues of sprouts this way: "Epidemiological studies indicate that to cut the risk of colon cancer in half, a person needs to eat about two pounds of broccoli and similar vegetables a week, a goal that few Americans meet. Given the chemical potency of broccoli sprouts, the scientists said, the same reduction in risk theoretically might be had with a weekly intake of just a little over an ounce of sprouts."

A medical science pioneer in the study of enzymes, the late Edward Howell, author of *Enzyme Nutrition*, identified enzyme shortages in the human body as being linked to such chronic illnesses as obesity, heart disease, certain types of cancer, and even premature aging.

When a human sperm and egg merge, it is enzyme activity that provides the spark for the formation of a new life. That spark is electric. It is lifeforce! At birth, we are each given a supply of enzymes that must be periodically renewed. As we age, our exposure to synthetic chemicals, our lifestyle habits, and, for most people, a steady infusion of foods subjected to high temperatures, depletes our storehouse of enzymes. Our backup system ought to be those enzymes derived from the food we eat, but if we are only eating cooked food, our enzyme resources will soon be exhausted. When this happens, the body puts out an emergency call for enzyme reinforcements to vacate the body's glands, muscles, nerves, and blood, and come to help in the demanding digestive process.

Raw, organic, living food will replenish that storehouse. That is another reason why we emphasize this enzyme-rich diet in the Hippocrates Program—we want our guests to be revitalized by the vitamins, minerals, proteins, and enzymes that support the body's immune system as the body detoxifies itself.

Supplemental enzymes designed by Dr. Howell give us a better way to digest our food and further expand our enzyme stores. When people use these supplemental enzymes, they experience a reduction in the symptoms of illness and an increase in energy. Additionally, more nutrients are absorbed into the human cell when supplemental enzymes are used to complement a proper diet. Supplemental enzymes will never be a replacement for raw living food, but they can help to improve our overall health.

While significant attention has been paid in the health literature to the beneficial role that digestive enzymes play in health mainte-nance, too little attention and credit have been given to the importance of food enzymes as the critical link between the con-sumption of raw food and the resulting health benefits. One of the key findings in experiments we have conducted at the Hippocrates Health Institute deserves highlighting to illustrate what I mean.

We have two basic understandings about digestive enzymes and food enzymes. One is based on the structure of these molecules and

avoiding amputation from diabetes

Since the age of sixty-five, I have had diabetes that resulted in four differ-ent surgeries to remove arteries from my left leg to replace damaged arteries in my right leg. In 2004, my vascular surgeon informed me that he might have to amputate my leg above the knee. My foot had sores that would not heal and the pain had become unbearable.

My two daughters, Nancy and Kara, had been to Hippocrates in 2002. Kara had a prolapsed colon and was scheduled for surgery, but after doing the Hip-pocrates Program she was able to cancel that surgery. My daughters arranged for me to do the program, and Nancy came along to assist me.

I arrived at Hippocrates in a wheelchair. They placed me on a raw food diet of fresh green juices, wheatgrass juice, and plenty of sprouts and salads. Within one day of being there, I saw the color of my leg and foot begin to change. It had been a reddish blue-black, and during the program it went back to 80 percent of its normal color. The swelling also disappeared, as did most of the pain.

By the second week, I was pushing my wheelchair around for exercise. I also found that I did not need to take my diabetes medicine, as my blood sugar level had stabilized. I am now eighty-one years old and feel I can lead a normal life. I know that the quality of my life has greatly improved.

ALICE BROWN
SEVIERVILLE, TENNESSEE

their ability to withstand the acidic environment of the stomach. The second is based on the advantages that enzymes bring to cellular function. After two decades of microscopic analysis of the cellular systems of thousands of people who have been guests at Hippocrates, we discovered and confirmed that digestive enzymes and enzymes found within plant foods clearly enhance the electrical frequency in and around cells of the body.

Enzymes are considered merely and only proteins by most nutritional scientists, whereas the work we have conducted using electron microscopes has revealed that all of the enzymes we cracked open contained electrical frequency. The outer shell of enzymes is a protein, just as the outer shell of the human body (the skin and red blood cells) is protein that is held together with protein fibrin. It would be just as incorrect to state from this information that the human body is protein alone as it would to infer that enzymes are protein alone. Furthermore, there is some evidence to support the idea that food enzymes begin to be assimilated as soon as they are in the human mouth, resulting in a transfer of electrical charge and absorption at this primary level well before they come in contact with the stomach. Discovering that the function of enzymes enhances the electromagnetic frequency of cells brings an entirely new and totally supportable science to the study of enzyme activity.

At Hippocrates, we have seen in practice, again and again, a simple biochemical truth—enzymes are at the heart of physiological healing. Our ancestors consumed an enzyme-rich diet. It was the nutritional basis of human creation. As a culture, we have wandered far from this simple yet profound biochemical truth.

The Hippocrates Program diet stops the waste of enzyme energy and makes daily deposits into the body's enzyme account. Few withdrawals and frequent large deposits are the key to being richly supplied with the metabolic enzymes that build, cleanse, and heal the human body.

animal proteins cause disease

After decades of biochemical and nutrition research and observation, T. Colin Campbell made a significant discovery. He found that nutrients, particularly protein, from animal-based foods increased tumor development, while nutrients and protein from plant-based foods decreased tumor development. "Dietary protein proved to be so powerful in its effect that we could turn on and turn off cancer growth simply by changing the level consumed," observes Campbell in *The China Study*, describing his laboratory experiments on cancer and nutrition.

The protein that most consistently stimulates cancer growth is casein, which constitutes 87 percent of the protein in cow's milk. The type of protein that does not promote cancer is only found in plants. People who eat the most animal foods are the unhealthiest of all categories of people based on diet, while people who eat a primarily plant-based diet are the healthiest of all. Children who eat the most animal protein, according to Dr. Campbell's findings, are at a significantly higher risk of developing liver cancer.

A casein/protein link to cancer was first identified in 1954 by a study published in the journal *Cancer Research*. This landmark study concluded that casein protein, as found in dairy foods, caused some forms of cancer to develop at a rate five times faster than average. Dr. Campbell expanded upon these findings in an experiment in which he found that casein increased cancer growth 100 percent of the time when it was introduced at any stage of cancer development.

The China Study shows the scientific research that supports the Hippocrates Program. We did the clinical research on people, and Dr. Campbell did the laboratory research. One of his most significant findings, in my view, is that dairy products have a higher correlation with tumor growth and lung cancer than does cigarette smoke. That is a revelatory finding supported by the most thorough research on nutrition ever done in history. It undermines most everything being taught in the biological sciences about human nutrition.

Many other common health ailments that plague humanity can be traced to animal proteins. W. G. Robertson of the Medical Research Council in Britain published a study in the *British Journal of Urology* demonstrating a direct connection between the formation of kidney stones and animal protein consumption. Professor Robertson healed his patients of recurrent kidney stones by shifting their diets away from all animal-protein foods.

Based on the results of hundreds of peer-reviewed medical studies, T. Colin Campbell was able to reach a series of dietary conclusions about the dangers of animal proteins versus the health benefits of plant proteins:

from Crohn's disease to healing

At age twenty, I was diagnosed with inflammatory bowel disease (IBD), also known as Crohn's disease and ulcerative colitis, a deadly affliction. The pain and suffering that come with this disease are intolerable. I felt an urgent need to have a bowel movement many times throughout the day without warning.

Upon receiving the IBD diagnosis, I was told that I was at high risk for colon cancer and to anticipate a lifelong relationship with this incurable malady. The physician's remedy was a barrage of prescription medications with horrific side effects. Feeling trapped, I searched endlessly for a way out, to no avail. This caused mental, emotional, and physical stresses that only increased the intensity of the disease. I was a mess and getting worse and worse.

After exhausting every available treatment (other than surgical removal of my colon, which doctors told me was the only true cure), I concluded that stress might be part of the cause. So thirteen years ago I left Wall Street and moved to South Florida. I adopted a vegan diet, and that, combined with my new locale, was of great assistance to my health.

Eventually, I participated in the three-week Hippocrates Program. I quickly became amazed at how these raw living foods that were healing me so rapidly were the same ones at the top of the list of foods that every doctor had advised me to avoid. I will never forget when I first arrived at Hippocrates and saw a lady walking very slowly with crutches, seeming very sick. Three weeks later, I did a double take when I spotted the same lady jogging. It was right then that I realized we should not live to eat but rather eat to live.

When I first started the program, I experienced ups and downs, but I made it through. The longer I lived this way, the easier it became. I have now been living the Hippocrates lifestyle for thirteen years, and it is so simple to me now that it's second nature. When I tell people about the program and the healing powers of raw living foods, they still badger me asking for proof. As I continually state, science fully supports this dietary choice, but my own experience of transformation from hopelessness to healing is far more convincing.

PAUL NISON
SOUTH FLORIDA

- Diabetic patients no longer need their medications if they abandon animal foods and adopt a plant-based diet.
- Dietary changes alone can reverse heart disease.
- Prostate cancer risk is greatly elevated by dairy food consumption.
- Consumption of animal-based foods raises the risk of women contracting breast cancer.
- Higher mental performance in old age is related to the antioxidants imparted from a diet reliant on fruits and vegetables.

Dr. Campbell's prescription for good health totally embraces the multiple health benefits of plant foods and the avoidance of all types of meat, eggs, and dairy foods. He states, "I did not begin with preconceived ideas, philosophical or otherwise, to prove the worth of plant-based diets. I started at the opposite end of the spectrum as a meat-loving dairy farmer in my personal life and an establishment scientist in my professional life. I even used to lament the views of vegetarians as I taught nutritional biochemistry to pre-med students."

Quite often, nutritional and medical researchers who have set out to try and debunk the health benefits of raw food have made discoveries totally at odds with their preconceived ideas. A 2005 study published in the *Archives of Internal Medicine* produced newspaper headlines: "Raw Food Vegetarians Have Low Bone Mass." But if anyone had bothered to actually read the study, they would have found that although those on a raw vegan diet did have lower bone mass compared to nonvegetarians, they also had high bone quality and *no* biological markers for osteoporosis, which is usually associated with low bone mass. Not only that, the raw food vegans had less inflammation and lower levels of IGF-1, which has been linked to a risk of breast cancer and prostate cancer. And in spite of the fact that the raw food group in this study did not drink milk or eat cheese, they had higher vitamin D levels than people on a typical Western meat-and-dairy diet.

The lead researcher for this study, which had been sponsored by the National Institutes of Health, Luigi Fontana, made this summary declaration about his findings: "If someone wishes to improve their health and reduce their risk of cardiovascular disease and cancer, I would definitely suggest that they get away from the refined and processed foods that Americans usually eat and try to eat a wide variety of nutrient-dense foods."

We also pay dearly for our ingestion of meat and animal by-products because of the many synthetic hormones, antibiotics, and other toxins these animals have been injected with and subjected to, and that we in turn absorb from them.

Raw plant food provides abundant protein for the human body's needs. Gorillas, elephants, and blue whales are just a few of the many powerful creatures whose protein sources consist exclusively of green foods. Many whole foods, such as spinach, contain more digestible protein than uncooked meat. Once meat has been cooked, its blood is no longer a source of essential amino acids, because its molecular structure has been permanently altered.

Here are some organic vegetable foods that contain the highest content of protein to meet human dietary needs:

ALGAE	
freshwater algae	sea algae
SPROUTED GRAINS AND GRASSES	
barley	oats
buckwheat	rye
corn	wheat
millet	wild rice (germinated)
SPROUTED LEGUMES	
black-eyed peas	lentils
broad beans	lima beans
fava beans	mung beans
Great Northern beans	navy beans
kidney beans	

the importance
of combining foods

Combining food in the most beneficial way for human health is a new science with two overriding principles:

1. Foods are chemicals, and combinations of chemicals produce different effects.
2. We all digest food at various rates in various acid and alkaline environments.

Our bodies are similar to a test tube in a chemistry laboratory. As with any chemistry experiment, depending on the combination of elements, we can create reactions ranging from sedative and healing to explosive and detrimental. The more synthetic chemical ingredients that are added to human-made supermarket products, the more opportunity people have to experience a digestive explosion and health problems.

By contrast, compelling evidence has emerged that certain combinations of raw vegetables and fruits can induce powerful healing synergies in the human body. Here are three examples from research studies cited by Karen Collins, a dietician and nutritional adviser to the American Institute for Cancer Research:

- **Broccoli and brussels sprouts.** Different phytonutrients in these two cancer-fighting vegetables combine when eaten together to stimulate phase-2 enzymes, substances known to prevent carcinogens from damaging human DNA.

- **Curcumin and quercetin.** The spice turmeric contains the phytonutrient curcumin, while quercetin is a phytonutrient found in yellow onions. When mixed together, these phytochemicals have been found to reduce the number of colon polyps in test subjects by 60 percent.

- **Oranges, apples, grapes, and blueberries.** Research has found that the antioxidants in these fruits, when combined in a meal, create effects much more powerful in eliminating free radical damage than any one fruit by itself.

Our digestive process is analogous to an automobile with varying levels of acceleration and speed. If we position a slow vehicle in front of a faster one on a one-lane road, the faster one must slow down to prevent an accident. In our digestive system, foods that digest more quickly crash into the foods that are digested more slowly, causing "accidents" in the form of indigestion, bloating, and poor assimilation of nutrients.

This principle has led us at Hippocrates to develop some basic food-combining groups and combinations that facilitate digestion

recovering from thyroid cancer

My health challenge began in December 1993, when doctors handed me their diagnosis of medullary thyroid carcinoma, a rare form of cancer of the thyroid gland. I was in shock. I was only thirty-four years old, with two beautiful children, eight and tens years old. Now my world was falling apart!

My doctors recommended a series of operations, because my case did not allow chemotherapy or radiation treatments. I underwent five operations over ten years, the last one leaving me with visible scars. Apart from the obvious scar on my neck, the sympathetic nerve was touched and the entire left side of my face was sagging. Modern medicine had clearly reached its limits at my expense.

Eventually, I decided to try the Hippocrates Program in Florida. All of the treatments I have since undergone there—the living food, the therapeutic juices, the regular and sustained exercises, the professional instruction—have enabled me not only to understand but also to integrate this lifestyle into my daily routine. As the saying goes, you are what you eat.

After the three-week program, my face regained its normal appearance (with the bonus of nicer skin), my energy level increased fivefold, and my metabolism stabilized. Today I eat consciously, because I am aware of all the benefits of this nutrition: increased levels of oxygen in my cells and more nutrients, vitamins, and enzymes to strengthen my immune system. After more than two years on this diet, my body, my mind, and my spirit are balanced, and I have gained health and inner peace.

MARLENE BOUDREAULT
QUEBEC, CANADA

and the assimilation of nutrients. These combinations are based on our many decades of experimentation and observation, noting how these various mixtures of foods affect the immune system response. For the best results, choose only the foods from a given group for each meal.

TABLE 4: *the four basic food-combining groups*

AVERAGE DIGESTION TIME	FOODS INCLUDED
FRUITS	
2 hours (for melons, 15 to 30 min.)	acids (grapefruits, lemons, oranges, pomegranates, and strawberries), sub-acids (apples, apricots, most berries, grapes, kiwis, mango, peaches, and pears), sweet (bananas, all dried fruit, and persimmons), and the melon family (canary, cantaloupe, Crenshaw, honeydew, Persian, Santa Claus, and watermelon)
PROTEINS	
4 hours	seeds (pumpkin, sesame, and sunflower) and nuts (almonds, Brazil nuts, pecans, pine nuts, and walnuts), but not peanuts or cashews
STARCHES	
3 hours	sprouted grains (amaranth, barley, millet, quinoa, rye, and teff), sprouted legumes (chickpeas, lentils, and peas), winter squashes (acorn, Hubbard, kabocha, and spaghetti), and sweet potatoes and yams
VEGETABLES	
2.5 hours	sprouted greens (alfalfa, arugula, buckwheat, cabbage, clover, garlic, kale, mustard, and radish), cruciferous vegetables (broccoli, cabbage, and cauliflower), vegetables (asparagus, celery, cucumber, fresh corn, red bell pepper, scallions, summer squash, and zucchini), leafy greens (arugula, bok choy, chard, collard greens, kale, lettuce, mizuna, mustard greens, spinach, and watercress), low-starch root vegetables (beets, burdock, carrots, parsnips, radishes, and turnips)

Two foods with excellent benefits when eaten alone are vine-ripened tomatoes, which cleanse the liver of deposited fats, and vine-ripened strawberries, which cleanse muscle and fat cells of waste materials. Nutritious combinations of foods are avocado and greens, avocado and sub-acid fruits, protein and sprouts with leafy greens, and starch and sprouts with vegetables.

Some poor combinations are fruit and starch together, fruit and vegetables together, fruit and protein together, starch and protein together, and starch and avocado. A typical mismatch in the Western diet is granola, which contains rolled oats (starch) and nuts (protein), combined with honey and dried fruits. Though tasty, it is a combination that creates various gasses in the body, including sulfur. The mixture of starch and sweet fruit creates fermentation and alcohol, neither of which is good for health.

the eighteen wonders of wheatgrass

n previous chapters of this book, a few of the many health benefits of wheatgrass have been described, but it would be useful to list them all to emphasize why this amazing plant is one of the cornerstones of the Hippocrates wellness program. To an untrained eye, the blades of wheatgrass may look similar to the blades of any common lawn grass. Wheatgrass is grown from the wheat berry, which is the whole kernel of the wheat grain, and the superior quality and variety of its nutrients are what set it apart from other grasses. Here are some facts about this amazing food.

Based on our research and observation, wheatgrass

- is one of the richest sources of vitamins A and C;
- contains a full, balanced spectrum of readily assimilated B vitamins, including laetrile (B_{17}), which has been credited with selectively destroying certain cancer cells without affecting normal cells;
- contains high-quality organic calcium, phosphorous, magnesium, sodium, and potassium in a balanced ratio;
- provides organic iron to the blood, which improves our circulation;
- contains 92 of the 102 trace minerals recognized as available in plants;
- is the most effective form of chlorophyll therapy;
- assists in reducing blood pressure;
- is similar to the chemical molecular structure of human red blood cells, thereby enhancing the blood's capacity to carry oxygen to every cell of the body;
- assists in eliminating drug deposits from the body;
- purifies the liver;
- helps wounds to heal faster;
- counteracts metabolic toxins in the body;

- combats blood sugar problems;
- has been credited with halting both hair loss and hair graying;
- aids in relieving constipation;
- increases resistance to radiation and eliminates the symptoms of radiation poisoning;
- acts as a disinfectant by killing bacteria in the blood, lymph, and tissues; and
- is considered a complete food because it contains all of the necessary amino acids for the human body.

Because wheatgrass acts as a powerful cleanser inside the human body, you may feel nauseous soon after ingesting it. This is a reaction to the release of toxins within your system. It is best to start with small quantities, one ounce or so, then gradually increase the intake to four ounces at a time. The same is true when using wheatgrass juice as an implant in the colon.

Once juiced, wheatgrass is not stable and tends to go rancid quickly. So it is best to drink it within fifteen minutes of juicing. However, cut grass will store for a week or so in a refrigerator if stored in a plastic bag or container. Frozen wheatgrass juice will keep for longer periods of time, though it is not as effective as freshly made juice, which has all of its nutrients intact.

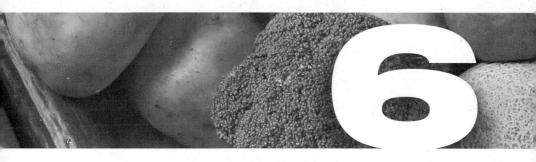

a pure food strategy for longevity

The art of healing comes from nature, not from the physician.

PARACELSUS, 1493–1542

If we could give every individual the right amount of nourishment and exercise, we would have found the safest way to health.

HIPPOCRATES

Every once in a while Hollywood succeeds at treating a profound subject in a serious and thought-provoking way. In the 2006 film *The Fountain*, the human desire for immortality, as symbolized by the quest for a fountain of youth, is portrayed in three time periods—the sixteenth century, the present time, and far into the future. The characters in each era find the answer to the secret of long life in the form of natural compounds from nature and by tapping into the lifeforce within our own human nature.

The search by medical scientists for a fountain of youth outside of nature and outside of our own bodies now consumes immense resources and inflates our imaginations with hollow promises. Entire industries have sprung up offering magic-bullet cures and quick fixes developed in laboratories, all in an attempt to convince us that science can extend our lives and eventually banish even the prospect of death, simply by tinkering with our body chemistry.

Early in human history, according to records of the time, we lived far longer, on average, than we do today. How was that possible? It is because we lived more in harmony with nature. The more we advanced technologically, the more removed we became from natural living. A return to longevity means a return to nature.

Aging should not be synonymous with illness, disease, infirmity, and a loss of mental agility. Longevity and good health are inextricably linked and are a recipe for happiness. After all, how happy can we be if we live to one hundred or beyond while painfully incapacitated by chronic ill health? As T. Colin Campbell puts it, "Good health is about being able to fully enjoy the time we do have. It is about being as functional as possible throughout our entire lives and avoiding crippling, painful, and lengthy battles with disease. The enjoyment of life, especially the second half of life, is greatly compromised if we can't see, if we can't think, if our kidneys don't work, or if our bones are broken or fragile."

Research on extending life-spans clearly demonstrates that the consumption of high-nutrient food in small amounts acts to prolong life by regenerating cells. A study published in the *Journal of the American Medical Association* in 2006 evaluated forty-eight people who were divided into four eating groups over six months and found that those on a low-calorie, high-nutrient diet had far more dramatic changes in metabolism and body chemistry, the sort of changes that have been linked to better health and a longer life.

Similarly, longevity research has produced a pattern of findings that show how animal products and cooked animal fats and proteins act to shorten life-spans. The science magazine *Nature* reported in 1974 that the more proteins laboratory animals ate, the shorter their life-spans became. An earlier study at the University of Helsinki in Finland found that all laboratory animals fed cooked fats died prematurely. As for humans, the results have been the same. A 1973 study, for instance, that appeared in the *American Journal of Clinical Nutrition*, revealed that the more animal fat a person eats the shorter that person's life-span will be.

We have also seen evidence emerge that some synthetic chemicals commonly added to foods may contribute to shortened life-spans. One is dihydrocoumarin (DHC), a chemical manufactured as a flavoring agent in a wide variety of foods, including soft drinks, yogurt, and muffins. It is especially concentrated in prepared gelatin, puddings, and frozen dairy products, and can even be found in many cosmetics and soaps.

In the online science journal *Public Library of Science Genetics*, a study was published in 2005 showing how DHC inhibits the activity of sirtuins, the enzymes associated with life-span control. During this laboratory experiment, DHC was injected into yeast cells; as a result, their life-spans were reduced by 30 percent. Yeasts contain many of the same sirtuins that humans have, and sirtuins have long been linked to aging and other important cellular functions, such as metabolism and neurodegeneration. Identifying which chemicals inhibit sirtuin functioning is an important step in making the case that synthetic food additives are a menace to human health.

At this point you may be asking yourself an obvious question: If most people are eating poorer quality food and their immune systems are under such a toxic assault from chemicals, why are we living longer, on average, than in the last few centuries? Average life expectancies for people in most industrialized countries increased by about forty years during the twentieth century. At the start of that century, people lived to their mid-forties on average; by the end of the century, people were living to their mid- to late seventies. Why did this happen and what does it mean?

An answer was provided by a 2006 report on health compiled for the American Society of Integrative Medical Practice by a group of physicians and scientists: "Improvements in hygiene, workplace safety, child labor, and waterborne illnesses have dramatically reduced fatal and maternal morbidity and mortality."

While overall life expectancy seemed to increase, despite a dramatic decline in the nutritional quality of the food available to most people, this statistical gain in longevity is exceedingly deceptive. As the research group of medical scientists also pointed out in their report: "When we compare the life expectancy of forty-year-olds in 1900 and 2000, there has been almost no change. More sobering, the current epidemics of obesity, hyperactivity, stress-related ills, stress fractures, and signs of early diabetes in our adolescents predict that in their twenties they will experience epidemics of full-blown diabetes followed, in their thirties, by cardiovascular, coronary, and cerebral diseases, poor fertility, and life expectancies many years shorter than their grandparents."

life extension with living food

At the age of thirteen, I had a mild case of pleurisy and was hospitalized. A young intern who decided to drain the fluid punctured my lung. Infection set in and I faced surgery, since there were no antibiotics at that time. My immune system was severely compromised, and it took me a year to recuperate. Life was never the same after that. I was plagued with fatigue, sleepless nights, and constant constipation.

Many years later, testing revealed that I had severe food allergies to milk protein, meat, cheese, and butter. At the age of seventy-four, I took a workshop by a Hippocrates health educator and living food lifestyle coach. That marked the beginning of my recovery. My diet become completely raw and organic.

Living food has given me boundless energy and a digestive system that now works properly and easily. It has also eliminated my constipation. At seventy-six years of age, I became an Iyengar yoga teacher. Now at age eighty, I teach yoga for seniors and live a high-quality life. The Hippocrates Program completely transformed me.

IDA ROBINSON
TORONTO, CANADA

Throughout human history people have been told what to "take" in ever greater quantities to help them live longer. The irony is that "taking" less actually creates greater health and longer life. For example, if we eat fewer calories, we will live longer. This principle extends to all aspects of our lives. The act of taking and draining ever greater quantities of the planet's resources, all for our own illusory creature comforts, is a form of consumer madness that not only diminishes our individual health and life-span, but puts the entire future survival and health of our species in jeopardy.

Nutrient deficiencies and lifeforce depletions, combined with the toxic chemical assault against our immune systems, will further reduce the life-spans of our children and grandchildren and inflict huge increases in health care costs on all of us. That process has already been set in motion and will accelerate, unless and until we begin to embrace more natural approaches to health and healing. It all begins with the lifeforce in our food and the lifeforce we regenerate within our bodies.

conquering the diseases of aging

You have probably heard this myth, and maybe you have even chosen to believe it—with age comes an inevitable decline in mental functioning. Not only is memory loss an unavoidable consequence of getting older, according to this myth, but Alzheimer's disease, the devastating illness that robs minds, chooses its victims at random and we are all at risk.

Like any myth based on fear and ignorance, this one ignores the evidence of both science and human experience. The mind and body can each be regenerated. This is one of nature's gifts of lifeforce. We have seen this truth in practice thousands of times with graduates of the Hippocrates Program, and these are results that medical science has verified in numerous ways.

Drinking fruit and vegetable juices can significantly reduce anyone's risk of developing Alzheimer's, a 2006 study in the *American Journal of Medicine* reported. A team of researchers at Vanderbilt University followed the health of nearly two thousand people over a decade and found the risk of Alzheimer's was 76 percent lower for persons who drank juice more than three times a week compared to study participants who drank it less than once a week. Both fruit and vegetable juices were included in the study.

Scientists suspect that the antioxidants in these juices "mop up" free radicals that damage body cells, and this process offers protection against the accumulation of clumps of beta-amyloid proteins in the brain, which are believed to be responsible for Alzheimer's. Fruit and vegetable juices may also make blood flow to the brain more efficient, since poor blood supply to the brain has been linked to the onset of the disease.

"Diet almost certainly plays a part in every person's Alzheimer's risk," commented Harriet Millward of Britain's Alzheimer's Research Trust. "Diet could offer a relatively inexpensive way to fight a disease that ruins countless lives and costs the NHS [the British health service agency] more than cancer, stroke, and heart disease put together."

Other studies have shown that diets high in vegetables and low in dairy and meat offer protection against dementia, which affects half of all Americans eighty-five and older. A 2006 report in the *Annals of Neurology* revealed how neurologists at Columbia University followed the health of two thousand elderly people in New York City and discovered that the participants who most closely followed a diet high in vegetables and low in dairy and meat had a 40 percent lower risk of developing Alzheimer's. Once again, the effect was attributed to the antioxidants in a plant-based diet.

Another study published that same year in the *Journal of Alzheimer's Disease* strengthened the hypothesis that dietary regimens involving a restriction of calorie intake can halt and even reverse Alzheimer's. Mount Sinai School of Medicine researchers tested the idea on two groups of squirrel monkeys—one group was fed a typical monkey diet, the other was given a diet 30 percent lower in calories. Not only were the amyloid protein levels associated with Alzheimer's affected by the reduced-calorie diet, but the diet increased longevity of a related protein called SIRT1, which is located in the same region of the brain that influences age-related diseases.

Phytonutrients, which are natural memory boosters and disease-protective compounds, are profuse in the Hippocrates Program diet. One of our favorites to use as a spice on food or as a supplement is turmeric, a curry spice whose active ingredient is curcumin. Neuroscientists who have studied the elderly in India have found a much lower incidence of Alzheimer's and colon cancer than in Western countries, and they attribute this primarily to turmeric, which has been a staple of Indian cuisine for an estimated five thousand years. Indian medicine has traditionally recommended it as an anti-inflammatory.

Only in recent years have Western scientists recognized the medicinal properties of this spice. *The Wall Street Journal* reported in 2005 that at least 256 science papers exploring the health benefits of curcumin had been published in the previous year, and the U.S. National Institutes of Health had initiated four clinical trials studying curcumin as a treatment for pancreatic cancer, multiple myeloma, Alzheimer's, and colorectal cancer.

Here are just a few of those research findings:

- A UCLA Veterans Affairs study found that curcumin may inhibit the accumulation of destructive beta-amyloids in the brains of Alzheimer's patients and might also break up existing plaques in those suffering from this disease.

- Yale University researchers discovered that curcumin helps to restore physiologically relevant levels of protein function in cases of cystic fibrosis.
- A November 2006 issue of the journal *Arthritis and Rheumatism* showed the effectiveness of curcumin in reducing joint inflammation and as a possible treatment for other symptoms of arthritis.

Fisetin is a naturally occurring flavonoid found in tomatoes, onions, strawberries, and other fruits and vegetables. Research published in the *Proceedings of the National Academy of Sciences* describes fisetin as a phytonutrient that stimulates signaling pathways in the brain in a way that enhances long-term memory. Fisetin was found to

overcoming breast cancer

During my last mammogram, the doctor found a small tumor that had not been there the previous year. Having been a medical professional for twenty years, I decided to seek second opinions from four other physicians. I had a biopsy and was diagnosed with infiltrating duct cell carcinoma.

A surgeon performed a lumpectomy and removed a few surrounding lymph nodes. I was subsequently referred to a radiation oncologist for follow-up treatment. At the time, my cousin from Barbados was visiting me and my husband. She told me, "You have already been invaded twice, and if you go further with this radiation, you will kill many healthy cells along with the cancer. You should go to the Hippocrates Health Institute."

Thanks to my cousin, I discovered a better way than more surgery and radiation. Hippocrates provided the perfect environment in which my mind and body could return to their natural state of health. After finishing the program, I maintained it at home and continued to heal myself. My surgeon confirmed my excellent condition and told me to continue whatever I was doing, as it was obviously working. She, like so many others, is now aware of all the benefits that I have received from the living food program.

LUCILLE BRADSHAW
ORLANDO, FLORIDA

protect and promote survival of neurons in the brain and to boost memory in mice that were tested with it in lab experiments.

Interestingly, a coauthor of the study, Pamela Maher, a researcher at the Cellular Neurobiology Laboratory at the Salk Institute for Biological Studies, pointed out that because fisetin is readily available in many foods in its natural state, there may be little financial interest for pharmaceutical companies and the medical industry to develop it as a treatment for memory loss associated with Alzheimer's and related diseases of aging. In other words, if these economic interests cannot patent a remedy such as curcumin or fisetin to protect their profits, they will not develop that treatment no matter how many lives will be saved and extended, or how much pain and misery will be avoided. This stark reality serves as a reminder that each of us is ultimately responsible for our own health and healing.

the secret of a long and healthy life

You have probably heard about the existence of certain isolated groups of people who live to one hundred years of age and beyond while remaining in good physical and mental health. One of these groups lives off the coast of Japan on the island of Okinawa and is among the most studied populations on the planet.

A saying carved into a stone beach marker in Okinawa reads, "At seventy you are but a child, at eighty you are merely a youth, and at ninety, if the ancestors invite you into heaven, ask them to wait until you are one hundred, and then you might consider it." That proverb reveals an attitude about living that helps to explain why the residents of Okinawa experience the longest disability-free life expectancy in the world.

Studies of the Okinawan diet reveal an emphasis on the consumption of dark green vegetables, sweet potatoes, bean sprouts, seaweed, onions, and green peppers. By contrast, meat, poultry, and dairy account for just 3 percent of their overall food consumption. With this diet fully ingrained into their lifestyle and culture, the rate of people living to one hundred years of age is six times higher than in the United States and other Western countries.

If you think the Okinawans may have a genetic predisposition toward longer lives, you would be wrong. When Okinawans leave the island and adopt the meat-and-dairy eating habits of other countries, they quickly fall prey to the same health problems that afflict the rest of the world's populations.

Harvard Medical School geriatrician Bradley J. Willcox, who spent a decade studying the food habits and lifestyle of Okinawa residents, cites four factors that account for their longevity: a low-calorie, plant-based diet, regular exercise, a strong spiritual tradition, and a positive outlook on life. "They are the happiest people I've ever seen," commented Dr. Willcox. When I read over his list of factors influencing life-span, it is clear that the Hippocrates Program, for over a half century, has been a successful embodiment of these principles in practice.

Another intensively studied group of people are members of the Seventh-Day Adventist Church in California, who adhere to a mostly vegetarian diet. A 2001 study in the *Archives of Internal Medicine* evaluated the health and diets of thirty-four thousand members of the church and found that those who ate the least amount of meat lived nearly ten years longer than those who regularly consumed animal products. Their incidence of disease in all categories was also significantly lower than meat eaters.

These findings have received broad support from other dietary studies for at least four decades. Two studies appearing in the *Journal of the American Medical Association* in 1961 and 1966, for instance, observed that people who do not eat meat live longer and suffer fewer chronic health disorders than meat eaters.

There is even scientific evidence for a correlation between IQ levels and good health. The *British Medical Journal* reported in one of its December 2006 online editions that children's IQ predicts their likelihood of becoming vegetarians as young adults, which in turn lowers their risk of developing cardiovascular disease later in life.

In this study, the British researchers collected data on 8,200 men and women aged thirty, all of whom had their IQs tested at the age of ten. Nearly 5 percent of these study participants were either vegan or vegetarian, and these individuals as a group had much higher IQ scores than the meat eaters.

"Brighter people tend to have healthier dietary habits," observed lead author Catharine Gale, a senior research fellow at the MRC Epidemiology Resource Centre of the University of Southampton. "This

beating cancer with diet

On New Year's Day 1995, I woke up with a lump the size of a big lemon on my neck. My wife insisted we go to the emergency room in Palm Springs, California, where we were vacationing. They took some blood tests and advised me to see my physician at home. My doctor diagnosed me with lymphoma (cancer of the lymph glands) and informed me that if I didn't immediately start chemotherapy treatments, I only had about six months to live. Even with those treatments, he said I could live for only another five years.

Our son-in-law, who is a certified nutritionist, suggested that I consider the Hippocrates Program. After a lot of reading, I decided it was my best bet. When I informed my oncologist, the pressure began. My general practitioner called me at home and tried to convince me that I was making a big mistake. So did my oncologist. My family and friends started getting on my case about not starting the treatments, so I caved in and began chemo. After my second treatment, my hair fell out and I looked like the walking dead. I decided that chemo would kill me before the cancer.

So I went to Hippocrates for a three-week visit in their program. I can truly say this has been one of the best decisions I have ever made in my life. Three years later, I am completely free of any cancer. I feel better and have more energy at age seventy-two than I did at age forty-two. I grow my own wheatgrass and sprouts and drink two quarts of raw organic vegetable juice every day. I spend a good deal of my time talking to people who want to find out what I did to defeat the cancer and to look so healthy.

BILL HUGHES
MODESTO, CALIFORNIA

study provides further evidence that people with a higher IQ tend to have a healthier lifestyle. Vegetarian diets are associated with lower cardiovascular disease risk in a number of studies, so these findings suggest that such a diet may help to explain why children or adolescents with a higher IQ have a lower risk of coronary heart disease as adults."

What is now indisputable are the reams of scientific studies demonstrating that meat eaters have shorter and more illness-plagued lives than their meat-free counterparts. When this IQ study was released, David Katz, the director of the Prevention Research Center at Yale University School of Medicine, told HealthDay News, "Studies, for example, of vegetarian Seventh-Day Adventists in California suggest that they have lower rates of almost all major chronic diseases and greater longevity than their omnivorous counterparts. Evidence is also strong and consistent that greater intelligence, higher education, and loftier social status—which tend to cluster with one another—also correlate with good health."

It is not just pure food but also pure water that helps to promote healing and a longer life-span. In 2000, we conducted a study among forty-six of our guests at Hippocrates to test the therapeutic impact of water harvested from a volcanically active area in Japan. This water, as measured by a gauss meter, contained a high electrical frequency charge. We invited twenty-three of our guests, all with catastrophic diseases and a bleak prognosis, to drink this water every day over a twenty-day period. We compared their progress with twenty-three other guests (also with similar ailments and a similar prognosis) who did not drink the volcanic water.

Those who drank the water, with its high electrical frequency, increased their immune system function by 18.5 percent on average, based on the findings of blood tests that we conducted. Absorbing the water had increased the electrons in their bodies to help shield red blood cells from decay. That lessened the burden on white blood cells, which in turn created greater immunity and an extended life-span.

Based on this study and other research we have conducted, longevity can be reduced to a basic formula: all physical and mental functioning operates on and through electrical frequency. To extend our lives, we must create a continuous wave of positive electrical activity. This means we need a constant infusion of the essence of life-force that comes from organic living food.

Life extension has become a big business, and at the center of this field is research into human growth hormones (HGH). Sometimes called somatotropin, HGH are hormones created in the anterior pituitary gland, which resides in the center of the brain. HGH produced by the pituitary gland is responsible for the body's growth, development, and regeneration. After the age of thirty, we experience a

TABLE 5: *24 foods to fight disease and extend your life*

FOOD	HEALTH-PROMOTING QUALITIES
Asparagus	When eaten raw, it provides the body with numerous minerals and phytonutrients. Research has shown it supports the kidneys and has a positive effect on emotions.
Black raspberries and blueberries	These two raw fruits provide an abundance of antioxidants, according to findings by the Tufts University Center on Aging. They help to reverse the harmful effects of aging on brain cells and may prevent Alzheimer's disease.
Cruciferous vegetables	Cabbage, broccoli, cauliflower, and brussels sprouts are rich in sulfur and help to fight cancer cells, reports the *Journal of Nutrition*. Consuming sprouted seeds of each vegetable increases the health benefits.
Daikon radish	When juiced, this Japanese root vegetable releases nutrients and phytochemicals to improve blood circulation, reduce ulcers, and assist the body with blood purification.
Endive	High levels of minerals and chlorophyll aid liver and blood detoxification and help the body to maintain vitality.
Fenugreek sprouts	Boost the gastrointestinal tract and have a positive impact on pancreatic blood sugar levels for sufferers of either high or low blood sugar.
Garlic	Researchers have found evidence the allyl sulfides in garlic inhibit the growth of cancer cells and help reduce ventricular plaque and inflammation, which are a cause of stroke and heart attacks.
Green pea sprouts	Due to their high beta-carotene content, these sprouts help to protect vision and create antioxidant effects against many forms of cancer. They also build muscle and healthy blood.
Hemp seeds and sprouts	This balanced food is rich in essential fatty acids and fuels a healthy metabolism by supporting the brain, organs, and nervous system.
Iceberg lettuce	While not usually known for its nutritional value, iceberg lettuce contains silica and silicon, which help to strengthen the skin, hair, bones, and nervous system sheath.
Jicama	Eaten raw or sprouted, it provides increased energy to the body while helping to maintain blood sugar levels and cardiovascular functioning.

Kale	High levels of calcium, phosphorous, and magnesium strengthen the teeth, skeleton, and red blood cells. Its sulfur content also helps with gastrointestinal disorders.
Lettuce	Leafy green varieties can elevate mood and increase sexual desire. Lettuce juice is often used as an aphrodisiac.
Mustard seeds (sprouted)	Clean mucous membranes and help to alleviate a wide range of respiratory disorders.
Nutmeg	A wide array of phytonutrients help to reduce bladder inflammation and decrease symptoms of frequent urination.
Onion	Its multitude of phytochemicals help to protect cells from mutagens as well as viral, fungal, and bacterial invaders.
Quinoa	Provides energy for mental and physical activity. Its high mineral and protein content help to alkalinize the body.
Red sweet peppers	Rich in vitamin C and other nutrients. Acts as an antioxidant to reduce free radical damage to cells and thus reduce the effects of aging.
Sweet potatoes	Along with their sprouted greens, they contain every vitamin and a majority of minerals and trace minerals. They increase vitality, strengthen the heart and other vital organs, and increase the ability of cells to regenerate.
Tomatoes	When organic and vine ripened, their phytonutrients help to prevent breast cancer and prostate cancer and strengthen the heart muscle.
Ugli fruit	Part of the grapefruit family, it contains citric acids, nutrients, and phytochemicals that dissolve wastes in the liver and gallbladder and create an antiseptic effect in the bloodstream. Also breaks up excess mucus in the body and reduces uric acid.
Watermelon	Along with its sprouted seeds, this fruit can flush the kidneys and bladder of impurities. When the outer skin is juiced, it provides high levels of protein and minerals.
Yucca	Along with its sprouted greens, yucca is commonly used as cleanser for the stomach and small intestine, and as a source of energy for physical activity.
Zucchini	Contains phytochemicals that may protect hearing and eyesight. Helps to reduce PMS and other female disorders. Its flowers provide high levels of beta-carotene, an important antioxidant for protecting the body from cancer and other diseases.

dramatic drop in the levels of these hormones, and as a consequence, according to much scientific research, this hormone deficiency becomes a central cause of aging.

Initially, as the antiaging field evolved, these growth hormones were extracted from pigs and then injected into people who could afford to pay the exorbitant cost of this procedure. The process of harvesting proved so challenging that the industry soon began using genetic modifications to create a stable source of supply. At Hippocrates, we have taken a strong stand against the use of genetically modified organisms because of the potential for toxic side effects. We have concluded that animal-based, chemically manufactured, and genetically modified products inherently create long-term negative consequences within the human body.

We do, however, recognize the need for naturally stimulating the pituitary gland to increase its production of human growth hormones. Hippocrates' research has affirmed the effectiveness of a natural HGH stimulator called atropine that retards aging. The natural chemistry of the pituitary gland is released by atropine. During a six-month experiment with our guests, we found that a majority of them reduced their weight, increased their stamina and sexual vitality, improved their memory and sleep regularity, and strengthened overall immune system function while using atropine.

For years we have taught that the true fountain of youth is to be found in pure, life-giving foods, regular exercise, positive thoughts, and a spiritual connection to the whole web of life. By naturally stimulating the body's production of HGH, we enhance the quality as well as the length of our lives.

As we age beyond forty, it is also more important than at any other stage of life to eat a mainly raw diet. A raw and living food diet is loaded with enzymes, vitamins, minerals, oxygen, and fiber. Living food, such as sprouts, which are still growing right up until the moment we eat them, provide us with a more subtle vitality, because the bioelectrical charge in these foods is at their strongest pitch.

Hippocrates' research experiments on the body's utilization of enzymes have produced evidence showing us how the infusion of fresh enzymes provides the human body with an enormous boost in improved digestion and healing at the cellular level. That is another reason that we recommend supplements in the form of whole food algae as a contribution to life extension.

Biochemist and Nobel Prize winner James B. Sumner of Cornell University says that the "getting old feeling" that many people report after the age of forty is a direct consequence of reduced enzyme levels throughout the body. Our young cells contain many hundreds more enzymes than our old cells, which become laden with metabolic wastes.

The word "enzyme" is derived from a Greek term meaning "to cause a change." That is exactly what enzymes do for the human body. They promote regenerative changes, which maintain health, protect against disease, and ensure longevity. They provide an energetic cellular charge, which is crucial to lifeforce. Food enzymes are essential nutrients to the human body that in their purest and most highly charged form can only come from raw organic food.

Over the past half century, there have been thousands of people who have gone through the Hippocrates Lifeforce Program after being given death sentences by Western medical practitioners. Many of these people are now in their nineties and beyond, and they are still flourishing, so we know our program works. We have seen its effectiveness in practice over the long term.

Longevity comes down to a very basic formula—all physical and mental functioning operates on and through electrical frequency. To extend our lives, we must work to create a continuous and unbroken wave of positive electrical activity in our thoughts and bodies. Simply put, we must find and embrace those activities, thoughts, and foods that charge us rather than drain us, and that empower us rather than enslave us.

The four cornerstones of the Hippocrates Program for a happy existence, good health, and a longer life are (1) life-giving thoughts, (2) emotionally satisfying connections with others, (3) life-giving food and exercise, and (4) and spiritual fulfillment.

herbs and supplements to keep your brain youthful

All of the following herbs and nutritional supplements should be consumed in their whole food form, which will ensure the complete and proper assimilation of all nutrient cofactors. Synthetic products in which nutrients are isolated in a laboratory do not provide the human body with all of the beneficial effects of supplements taken directly from whole food sources. For more information on medicinal herbs, see Chapter 14.

- **Alpha-lipoic acid** is a molecule that activates glutathione, a powerful antioxidant in our cells, and this in turn stimulates our ability to neutralize the free radicals that damage brain neurons.

- **B-complex vitamins** benefit our nervous system, help our brain to sustain the activity of neurotransmitters, and are important to overall mental and cardiovascular functioning. Deficiencies of these vitamins may result in depression, dementia, and nerve degeneration.

- **Blue-green algae** is a superfood by any standard. It has a high protein content (50 percent), which makes it helpful for alleviating depression. For longevity and mental function in particular, try Klamath Blue-Green Algae's alcohol-free Brain Power tincture, which also contains ginkgo leaves and other herbs.

- **Cat's claw** is a plant from South America that helps to prevent or counteract attention deficit disorder (ADD) in children and dementia in adults.

- **Coenzyme Q10** (CoQ10) is an essential enzyme and antioxidant within our body cells that helps to convert oxygen into usable energy. It also helps to protect neurons and other cells from mutating to create memory loss, dementia, senility, and Alzheimer's disease.

- **DHEA,** derived from wild yam extract, is a beneficial steroid that helps to prevent the deterioration of brain cells by producing the hormones estrogen and testosterone.

- **Hemp seeds** that are germinated produce usable omega-3 and omega-6 fatty acids, which help to nourish and rebuild brain structure.

- **Kava** is an herbal extract that reinvigorates brain cells to counteract depression and melancholia.

- **Melatonin** is a hormone that, with periodic use, helps to counteract sleep deprivation caused by premature or unnatural aging. It may also disrupt the enzyme functioning of the liver and gallbladder, so it should be used only sparingly and under the supervision of a competent and sympathetic health practitioner.

- **Memory foods** are those that have been identified as having a protective antioxidant benefit for enhancing human memory.

doctors stunned by recovery

When I entered the Hippocrates Program in July 2005, I weighed 243 pounds, my heaviest weight ever. I was fifty-three years old and had been a diabetic for three years. My cholesterol was out of control, and I had kidney stones. My prostate had some calcification, and I felt sluggish and tired all of the time. My physicians only wanted to prescribe more drugs. I was feeling desperate.

I decided to enter the Hippocrates Program. After a few weeks there, something amazing happened! It was like I had passed through an invisible barrier and had come out on the other side. I began to feel like my body had been born again. I reached a level of health that I had never felt before, merely by going from eating a standard North American diet to living on fresh, raw, organic vegetation.

In the year since my visit, I lost forty-four pounds and still lose about a pound a week. Both my family doctor and my urologist are amazed at my good physical condition. My glucose and cholesterol readings are both in the normal range. My urologist, who has followed me for twenty years, was sure there was a mistake when he took my X-rays. There were no traces of kidney stones anymore, and my uric acid level had returned to normal.

Today I am very much at peace and feel energized. The pleasure of conventional and junk food is incredibly small compared to the pleasure of my new sense of health. I am glowing and high with energy. I am running, skiing, and training effortlessly five or six days a week, activities that I never dreamed I would be able to do again.

MICHEL BEAUDRY, MONTREAL
CANADA

They include artichokes, beans, blackberries, blueberries, cinnamon, cloves, cranberries, hazelnuts, oregano, pecans, sweet potatoes, and walnuts.

- **Noni,** a fruit native to the South Pacific, has a unique chemistry that enables it to regenerate the receptor points in our cells, helping to forestall the degeneration of brain cells.

- **Oxygen** nourishes the brain and intensifies brain function. There are many effective forms of supplemental oxygen.

- **Phycomin**, which is rich in phytochemicals, is an extract of blue-green algae and acts to counteract depressive disorders and combat patterns of counterproductive brain chemistry.

- **Rutin**, a member of the B-vitamin family, helps to stimulate healthy circulation in all parts of the body, especially the brain.

- **Seawater** nourishes and reinvigorates, because its chemical composition is similar to that of human blood.

- **Vitamins C and E**, when consumed in combination in whole food supplement form, protect brain neurons from free radicals and can reduce or eliminate attention deficit disorder. They also act in concert as a potent, natural anticoagulant to facilitate blood flow throughout the body.

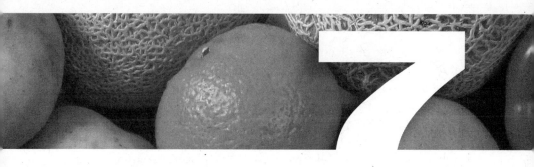

from a lead to
a platinum lifestyle

*Healing is a matter of time, but it is
sometimes also a matter of opportunity.*

HIPPOCRATES

We have all sometimes felt or have observed in others the symptoms of a "lead" lifestyle. It is evident when we rely on a diet of fast food, processed food, and meat and dairy products. It is a sedentary lifestyle that produces toxic bodies and quite often toxic minds and toxic thoughts.

For anyone to become a modern alchemist and transform a lead lifestyle into a platinum one, the highest level of a sustainable diet and health, requires a commitment to a constructive belief system. Our beliefs represent the totality of who we are and what we aspire to be. The foundation of any positive belief system is our self-esteem.

There are platinum levels of health and exercise and lead levels of lethargy and laziness. There are platinum levels of nutritious, health-promoting food and lead levels of toxic, disease-causing food. There are platinum levels of integrity and honesty and lead levels of self-deceit and chronic denial.

Your degree of success at transforming your life from lead to platinum will depend on the depth of your self-esteem. Do you have integrity? Are you honest with yourself and with others at all times? Do you feel worthy of other people's trust? Are you someone who keeps promises? Is your word as good as gold?

No one is entirely immune to the psychological attachments of former eating habits. Our first steps on the platinum path are usually baby steps. But those first steps must include the elimination of addictions to coffee, sugar, smoking, alcohol, and drugs, which are substances that keep the body in a perpetual state of toxic shock.

Rarely does anyone make quantum leaps on this path. Transformation is usually more like the change of seasons—gradual, definitive, and steady. Your obligation to yourself is to establish a goal, proceed to that goal with determination, embrace the goal upon reaching it, and then establish a new and higher goal. You can be sure that you are on track when your new companions are healthful eating habits, heightened self-esteem, happiness, and an enlightened spirit.

If you eliminated only 8 percent of the toxic parts of your diet each month, by the end of a year you would be living a positive, platinum-level life. In reality, it is usually an evolution that takes most people decades to complete. After you have eliminated the toxic addictions from your life, set this three-step process as a goal:

- **Step one:** Eat only organic food. The elimination of pesticides and other synthetic chemicals from your diet is a necessary part of this process.

- **Step two:** Reduce or eliminate your consumption of meat and dairy products. Create an action plan and stick to it.

- **Step three:** Reduce or eliminate your consumption of cooked food. Gradually eat larger and larger salads and greater quantities of raw food and vegetable juices.

It is important to recognize and take into account our individual differences and age when we consider our metabolism. As we age, our metabolism slows down; that is a fact of life. People in their teens and twenties have a much easier time metabolizing cooked food than do older people. Thus, if we are older, we will benefit even more from a commitment to a platinum diet and lifestyle.

Each of us can and should individualize the Hippocrates Lifeforce Program to gain the greatest benefit from it. Since you can choose among five tiers (excluding lead, which is a starting point rather than a place to go), choose the level at which you are likely to succeed and flourish.

The five tiers from highest to lowest are platinum, gold, silver, bronze, and copper. Ideally, each person should achieve and maintain the highest level possible. We should always be aware that no one is fixed at any given level but can—and should—aspire to a higher one. Even if you are perched on the platinum plateau, try to refine your habits further and sustain yourself at that level.

platinum. This is the highest level, where we utilize the most self-replenishing fuel to maintain our life at peak performance. People who have great responsibility, are competitive athletes, or who simply desire the highest level of awareness and functioning should strive to live in this energized way. At this pinnacle, you consume 100 percent organic, vegan living food, exercise aerobically for a minimum of one hour five days a week, do resistance exercise for at least ninety minutes three days a week, and undertake some form of daily spiritual self-development.

Local and/or global community contribution becomes a part of your weekly schedule, and you have appropriate rest and harmonious interaction with nature and life. Those who are in the process of recovery from catastrophic disease or illness must nevertheless strive to maintain the platinum paradigm. By employing and maintaining this level of integrity, you will achieve and sustain greater insight, awareness, health, and functioning. In addition, your elevated body and brain chemistries will compel you to fulfill your greatest aspirations and will open ever wider vistas to your unlimited potential and potency.

The respected actor and humanitarian Dennis Weaver (the star of TV's *Gunsmoke* and *McCloud*) and his wife Gerry adopted the Hippocrates Lifeforce Program decades ago. Because of their demanding schedules and committed social agendas, the program greatly benefited their personal and global activities and causes. They contributed to the welfare and future of humanity and the environment well into their golden years.

gold. The gold level is one step beneath platinum. Those who function in positions of authority that entail considerable responsibility, people at the early stages of legitimate aspirations, and those engaged in frequent but purely recreational athletics thrive at this level. They perform aerobic exercises five days a week for at least thirty-five minutes a day and resistance exercises for a minimum of forty-five minutes a day three times a week. They engage in spiritual self-development at least every other day, and their diet consists of approximately 80 percent living, organic, vegetarian food, and as much as 20 percent organic vegan cooked food.

On the gold tier, community and/or global contribution should be part of a monthly schedule, and appropriate rest and interaction with nature and the ecology are required. People with slightly less active lives thrive at the gold level; it is also suitable for those with less extreme health problems and life challenges.

silver. This is usually the entry level for those interested in improving their health and expanding their horizons. They are not facing imminent illness, and they have the time and interest to move slowly but surely up the ladder to a more refined lifestyle. Many retired people are at the silver level, as well as those with practical but limited ambitions. Exercise hobbyists who have a general interest in personal growth may start or function at this level. Their diet is 100 percent organic and vegan, and consists of as much as 40 percent cooked food and 60 percent living food.

People at this level do occasional aerobic and resistance exercise for a minimum of three days per week for at least twenty to thirty minutes each time. The silver tier requires at least one or two days of personal development each week and a minimum of one hour each month of local and/or global contributory efforts. Since this is the middle level, people in middle management might be found here as well as those in the middle of their careers and those in the midst of personal, familial, professional, and minimal medical challenges.

Not long ago, Tom Kelly was sent by his wife—a long time vegetarian—to experience the Hippocrates Program. He was under considerable work-related stress, had been gaining weight, and was lethargic and apathetic. Although he had an organic vegetarian diet at home, he would often sneak some dairy foods and conventionally prepared, pesticide-riddled fruit and vegetables when he went out for lunch at work. Then in his fifties, he wanted to renew himself and improve his life. He called himself a realist who did not aspire either to consuming much raw living food or to regular exercise. His life was so predictable that he rarely looked beyond his own limitations to consider the greater sphere.

When we suggested that Tom spend time in significant reflection every day, his first response was, "I can do this on weekends." He was, however, willing to live in a better way if he could do so without complete personal commitment. Despite this limited commitment, Tom lost thirty-five pounds and lives a much less stressful and more fulfilling life. Despite Tom's self-imposed limits, his health, attitude, and functioning have significantly improved, and as a result of this improvement, Tom now intends to move to the next level and beyond.

bronze. Newcomers usually start at the bronze level because it is the entry level. People who feel trapped in conventional modes of living function but do not flourish at this stage, because although it is less challenging, it is also less rewarding than the higher plateaus. Those who have minimal activity and motivation tend to be attracted to the bronze lifestyle. It requires a diet of only 40 percent living food, with the inclusion of as much as 60 percent cooked vegan food. People at this level attempt to consume organic food but are not always successful in doing so. Bronze living requires aerobic and resistant exercise for twenty to thirty minutes at least two days a week and some interest in individual growth and global awareness. Newcomers to a positive mind-set and people dealing with minor health issues often use this phase as the first step toward significant personal development. You should not expect to maintain anything other than average health if you remain at the bronze level, because it is a low-test fuel, not a premium one.

Sara Stone, who had recently lost her husband, was confronting the early stages of arthritis and menopause. She attended the Institute half heartedly and only at the behest and in the company of her son. Throughout her time with us, Sara joked about all the junk food she had always eaten. She even threatened to sneak out at night to indulge her junk food craving. Her symptoms of menopause and arthritis vanished less than three months after she completed our program. But Sara slowly regressed from a mostly raw organic diet to a mostly cooked one. Consequently, although her disorders were controlled, she would often be awakened by the painful stiffness of her joints. Only when her arthritis became a significant concern would she revert to living food, struggling for years with her dependency on cooked food. Eventually she was able to eliminate it and is now in total health and functioning at the gold and even platinum heights.

copper. People at the copper level face a broad horizon of improvement. They are influenced by family, friends, media, and other external forces. Their interest in health and self-development has been minimal, and they are not motivated to improve their circumstances despite the fact that often those circumstances are neither of their own making or choosing. Although they are vegetarians, their diet often includes as much as 20 percent dairy products and 80 percent vegan fare, with minimal or no emphasis on raw living food. People at this level typically consume nonorganic food, and they manifest neither effort nor interest in improving their diets. They rarely exercise regularly. Usually they are unaware of the world beyond their own insular reality, and so they are rarely involved in any service to their fellow beings and their world.

Lee Rush awoke with a pain shooting down his left arm. When the emergency medical team pronounced him healthy, his concerned neighbors, who had thrived on the Hippocrates Lifeforce Program, suggested that Lee and his wife Sally visit the Hippocrates Health Institute. Sally's gentleness and common sense allowed her to adapt to the life change well. Lee struggled with it from the beginning but maintained it in his own limited way. At home, friends often tell Lee that he eats like a rabbit, which too often causes him to compromise his commitment to healthy living. Although he has had no other health-related alarms and is now a vegetarian (in contrast to his former diet, which included considerable meat consumption), he has not yet found the personal resources to allow him to embrace higher levels of health and functioning. Even at the copper level, however, he has come far enough to have hopes of advancing further.

Those who are not on any of the five tiers are still eating animal-based food, which threatens their health and the planet's existence. Also stuck in this sand trap are people who do not exercise at all—80 percent of contemporary humanity—and who have no vitalized spiritual dimension, lack any interest in the world beyond themselves, and are forced by both external and self-imposed limitations to the point where they cannot, at least for now, imagine any way out of their plight.

Certainly there are many people who have a combination of some but not all of the deficiencies mentioned above. Many people who are devoted to exercise but eat animal products may appear in robust health, but they are degenerating internally. Others might have a relatively nutritious diet but are self-restrictive to the point of excluding human interaction and nature from their personal sphere. Still others focus exclusively on spirituality while excluding a wholesome diet, exercise, nature, and positive interaction with others.

This is not to say that people who are mired in the sand are permanently stuck there. Many people I know can attest to former self-indulgent diets, minimal or inappropriate exercise, self-imposed lack of interaction, limited or inappropriate interactions with nature, minimal service to our communities, a dearth of spirituality, and many other unwise choices. But, like many of you who may be reading this book and currently feel trapped in quicksand, they recognized what needed to be done and elevated themselves to the higher tiers.

People may appear to thrive within a broad range of living habits. As deceptive as these modes of functioning may be, particularly at the lowest ranges, the power of a positive attitude often allows people to inspire their body, mind, and emotions far beyond the limited energy imposed by improper living. Amazingly, the consumption of meat and dairy products, which we now know negatively affects human health in extremely severe ways, is still a topic of discussion by quasi authorities who themselves struggle against—and suffer from—their own established habits.

Given their amazing dynamism and adaptability, people often function, or appear to do so, despite blatant abuse of their own health, be it mental, physical, emotional, spiritual, or any combination of these. We use food as a diversion from consciousness rather than for its intended purpose of establishing and maintaining our health. Drugs, including such toxic stimulants as nicotine, caffeine, and alcohol, are other commonly used means of reducing awareness in order to hide from life and responsibility. Because we all know this at some level, we should strive to function at the highest possible tier at all times.

All five tiers encompass entire modes of functioning and can be personally established as masterpieces of artful, improved living. But we can still use refinement and balance on every plateau. Platinum might be implemented by either the moderate or the concerted approach. Asian medicine established balance by the paradigm of yin and yang; and the Hippocrates Program elevates it to a very different plane.

The consumption of nuts, seeds, avocados, and other foods containing high amounts of oil produces a slower metabolism and reduced awareness. Eating large amounts of fruit stimulates blood, electrical circulation, and hormonal brain activity, which sometimes cause a loss of mental focus as well as physical and emotional strength. Including significant amounts of germinated green food in your diet will allow you to attain heightened levels of efficiency and functioning without the overstimulation caused by fruit, which contains significant quantities of sugar and water.

Most of those who prevail at the platinum peak, strengthening their immune systems and elevating their functioning, nevertheless occasionally revert to the gold level. When one is dealing with an intense situation or severe negativity, the higher plateaus achieved with the platinum's superior electrically charged diet, exercise, and attitude

healing hepatitis with living food

As a young lady in my twenties, I found myself constantly exhausted. I was so tired I could not even brush my hair, because I could not lift my arms. When I went to the doctors they found a low-grade fever and put me into the hospital for a liver biopsy. From that I was diagnosed as having hepatitis C. They told me it was chronic and persistent, and of course they offered no help, telling me the only thing I could do was rest.

Concerned friends told me I must make sure that my diet was organic. To me that meant eating organic meat, fish, and poultry. The doctors were concerned about my hepatitis and suggested that I take interferon, at a yearly cost of $30,000, which was covered by my insurance. But, in their own words, taking it would not be of any permanent help.

I had to do something, so I began acupuncture and Traditional Chinese Medicine. This made me feel slightly better, but not as well as I needed. Finally, I found an alternative physician, Anthony Bazzan, from Jeffersonville, Pennyslvania, and I began to work with him. When he saw my viral load count he was shocked. It was double what it had been just months before. My liver enzymes were always high over the last few decades, and they certainly had not improved. When Dr. Bazzan asked me what I was eating, I expected him to congratulate me when I described my organic steamed vegetables and fish, but he told me it was processes do not permit a comfort level that will accommodate lesser involvement. After significant initial refinement of the body/mind, the gold tier is apparently the easiest level at which to maintain that refinement in this high-speed, polluted, stress-inducing world.

This framework for improved living is a map that guides you to ever higher peaks of personal fulfillment and self-refinement. This is not a judgment but a statement of fact. Since contemporary living is often difficult and stressful, considerable latitude must be given to those who are seeking to improve their lives and consistently progress in their pursuits. Since we are climbing a figurative mountain that feels quite real, we must also have the courage to pick ourselves up and dust ourselves off after the occasional temporary fall.

all wrong. He told me I needed to be on all raw food, and he strongly suggested that I attend the Hippocrates Health Institute.

I began eating a raw food diet. It was hard to do this on my own. I started to go to a local woman who grew wheatgrass, and I bought a juicer and began mixing this remarkable elixir shortly after I enrolled in the three-week program at Hippocrates. Going to Hippocrates was one of the highlights of my entire life. I learned how to take responsibility for every aspect of my life and health. By doing so, I was absolutely healed.

For the first time since I was a young lady, my liver enzymes became normal and my energy level rose to such a degree that I even surprise myself. Before I went to Hippocrates, my body was bloated and I was always hungry. I used to have to eat every two hours. As an added bonus, on the living food diet I have lost twenty-five pounds.

I cannot suggest strongly enough for those of you suffering with what medicine calls a catastrophic disease, such as hepatitis, to adapt and enjoy the living food lifestyle. Of course, you must persevere, because the only way that we can recover from our disease is by taking personal responsibility for our health. I've found something I had been seeking for so long, and it was so simple, not complicated, and right there all of the time.

KAREN HARKINS
WEST PALM BEACH, FLORIDA

Do not think of yourself as a habitual failure; know yourself as a consistent success. Your ability to maintain an integrity-rich existence will not be determined by a snapshot of you climbing up a steep hill; instead, it will be the epic motion picture that represents your successful climb to life's highest levels.

The high-test fuels of specialization and separation have revved the hot rod of the nutrition business into overdrive. We are being purposely confused by the notion that each of us needs a uniquely individualized diet. But in addition to the essential nutrients listed in Table 3, every healthy body requires only HOPE—hormones, oxygen, phytochemicals, and enzymes—and this can be achieved only by the consumption of raw living food.

Our diminished health often becomes so ordinary to us that the startlingly healthy increase in our energy and vision fueled by HOPE can initially create some discomfort. It is a little like taming a horse: This proud, beautiful creature gets riled when you swing onto his bare back and try to ride him. If, however, you calmly and gradually earn his trust, he will become not only responsive but cooperative. Entering a new way of living is the same as riding that wild horse: As you establish trust and faith, your task becomes fulfilling and rewarding. While you should not saddle yourself with guilt and unreasonable expectation, you should spur yourself to ride toward your objective just as comfortably and quickly as you can.

rediscovering an ancient truth

A specialist in nutritional anthropology, H. Leon Abrams, who teaches anthropology and sociology at the University of Georgia, studied the scientific research of paleontologists and discovered that the use of fire to prepare food began about ten thousand years ago with the advent of agriculture. Prior to that time, humans were hunter-gatherers who ate mostly plants found in their natural state in the wild. "The remains of human skeletons from the Paleolithic era," writes Professor Abrams in his foreword to the book *Raw Food Nutrition*, "show that these people had practically no dental decay and that they were in exceptionally good health. Their diet was obviously particularly healthy."

As humans domesticated animals and became dependent on the growing and consumption of cereal crops, humanity's health began to deteriorate under an onslaught of degenerative diseases. The lesson for us today is clear. "Our Paleolithic ancestors ate a great variety of natural raw foods, without altering them, and they apparently lived in good health on this diet, which remained practically unchanged during the three or four million years of humanity's development," continues Professor Abrams.

"As a result of our hunter-gatherer origins, and because human genetics evolve very slowly, the natural raw diet of our ancestors is undoubtedly the most ecological today, still perfectly adapted to the human species. Modern scientific knowledge in the fields of anthropology and nutrition show that we can live better, easily achieve better health, and halt the current process of degeneration of the species, simply by adopting a raw natural diet."

In our work with the Hippocrates Lifeforce Program, the use of raw and living food has evolved into a way of living and eating that forges a new relationship between food and life. This relationship is not a novel concept; rather, it is a reemergence of an ancient truth. Germinating and sprouting food, using grasses and leafy green vegetables, understanding the importance of juices, and the careful inclusion of some dehydrated and fermented foods are the keys to this reemergence.

Many ancient cultures knew the value of germinating and sprouting grains, seeds, legumes, and nuts. The use of sprouted seeds for food and medicine is more than twice as old as the Great Wall of China and was even noted in Chinese historical records. Today, more and more data is being compiled on the amazing nutritional value of sprouts.

Living food that is germinated and sprouted affords us the most concentrated natural source of vitamins, chelated minerals, enzymes, and amino acids. It also contains abundant enzymes and bioelectrical energy, making it highly desirable. Pound for pound, lentils and other bean sprouts contain as much protein as red meat, yet in a digestible form without the fat, cholesterol, hormones, and antibiotics that are found in meat.

Germination is the important process that results when seeds, grains, legumes, and nuts are soaked in water for a period of time. Water removes certain metabolic inhibitors, which are present to protect the seed from bacterial invasion and preserve it during its dormant state. Soaked seeds are more easily digested. During the germination process, the seed springs into life and its nutrition becomes more readily available to us. Germination is the process employed to make many of the seed and nut sauces at the Hippocrates Health Institute and is

overcoming a rare disease with wheatgrass

About eleven months ago, I began to feel rather nauseated, and I had no idea why. I could not eat without having the sensation to vomit, and I felt extremely fatigued after exercising (this was the least of my symptoms). A couple of weeks later, I got a weird rushing sensation throughout my whole body, and I felt like I was chemically out of balance. This really freaked me out and caused me go to the doctor, where I got the expected response, "It looks like a bit of an anxiety problem, but we will get a blood test to be certain." I had never experienced such anxiety attacks before in my life. Once the blood results were returned, I was diagnosed with Gilbert's syndrome, which is a liver condition (my bilirubin levels were high). Doctors labeled this as a benign disorder, yet I was left perplexed at living with such annoying symptoms.

After being hospitalized five times, the doctors still told me that Gilbert's syndrome was nothing to worry about. This struck me as ironic, since I was experiencing severe anxiety attacks and heart palpitations, not to mention the accompanying depression, joint pain, muscular discomfort, extreme fatigue, poor memory, nausea (which led to anorexic-like symptoms due to being unable to eat), terrible headaches, irritable bowel, low body temperature, and an overall toxic feeling. Once I detailed all of this again for the physicians, they thought I had something more serious, perhaps chronic fatigue syndrome. I realized I was becoming a hypochondriac. I was developing into an agoraphobic home dweller who had reached his retirement at the age of thirty!

I couldn't go anywhere without the sensation that I was going to die and help was not at hand. The doctors continued giving me prescription after prescription to help me with the multifaceted discomforts and depression. Since my liver was already malfunctioning, the drugs only served to worsen my condition. My liver was only producing enzymes at 30 percent of the normal rate, and my body was riddled with toxins, which were wreaking havoc. I learned that my joint pain was due to the toxic buildup, which was giving me arthritis-like sensations.

In search of a solution, I began to change my diet, and I noticed a smidgeon of relief. I could not consume any fatty food without vomiting (perhaps this was a blessing in disguise). I tried one product after another from health shops, as I continued to see new physicians in pursuit of something to alleviate the drudgery of living. Striving to exercise my body daily was a tough pill to swallow, as I would feel knackered from just fifteen minutes of walking. I was not only a physical wreck but an emotional one.

Then I discovered an organic shop in New Zealand, where I was advised to take a shot of wheatgrass each day. I was bewildered by this, as I only associated this kind of thing with grazing animals. But I was desperate enough to try almost anything at this point. The first day I took it I felt absolutely horrible; I was bedridden. Oddly enough, the next day I felt okay. After taking it for three days, I perceived a difference when I went for my usual fifteen-minute walk (all I could previously muster) and noticed I wasn't feeling tired. Two days later, I felt like never before; I was rather energetic. I thought some sort of a miracle had happened, but no, the wheatgrass had helped my body to get to the correct nutritional balance, just as my liver had thrown it out of whack. I couldn't believe it! I felt like I had been reborn!

I had such zeal that I recommended wheatgrass to a friend who was born with a degenerative condition and had only one kidney. Nearing dialysis, he took it habitually, and what do you know—his blood pressure normalized; something that had not been achieved with his medication.

I now heartily believe in consuming wheatgrass, and I desire to share its wonders with others. Upon learning that the Hippocrates Health Institute utilizes wheatgrass as an integral component of their program, I contacted them with my story so that I could do my part in spreading the word to others who may be suffering as I had been.

EMILIO MORALES
CANARY ISLANDS

also the first step in the sprouting process. Sprouting carries this life-beginning process further, resulting in a variety of living food.

In our research, we have concluded that while there are virtually endless varieties of food that can be sprouted, the most beneficial sprouts provide for different types of utilization by the body. Wheatgrass and tray-grown greens provide chlorophyll, and they clean and rebuild the body most efficiently. The next group of efficient greens includes alfalfa, clover, radish, cabbage, daikon, chia, and broccoli. The energy givers are the grains, which include wheat, oats, rye, barley, and buckwheat, and the legumes, which include pinto, navy, red, and white beans. Mung and adzuki beans also provide important minerals, and fenugreek seeds should be added for improved digestion and elimination.

It is a fact that today we are reexamining the foods we eat and going back to the ancient truths of proper diet through living food. The health benefits we get from this inexpensive, abundant, and nutritious food are the ideal way to combat the modern-day problems of dietary deficiency and the only way to combat world hunger for the long term.

rating the lifeforce energy in our food

Over the past few decades, we at Hippocrates have conducted research into the electrical frequency of our food and the effect that electrical charge has on the frequency of healthy cells. In conjunction with the photographic research conducted at UCLA in the mid-seventies, which measured the relative energy level in different foods, we have created a list of foods from highest to lowest in energy content.

Why are wheatgrass, edible weeds, and tropical fruits at the top of the list? Because they have the most sunlight, or lifeforce energy, in them. In this system, we recognize that all life on the planet comes

TABLE 6: *five-star foods* $*****$

TYPE OF FOOD	EXAMPLES
Algae (blue-green; freshwater)	—
Algae (green; freshwater)	chlorella
Fruit, tropical (ripe, organic)	mango, papaya, pineapple, star fruit
Plants, baby (sprouted)	buckwheat, fava bean greens, peas, sunflower, sweet potato greens, wheatgrass
Sea vegetables	arame, dulse, hijiki, nori, Pacific or Atlantic kelp
Weeds, edible	chicory, dandelion, lamb's-quarters, plantain, purslane

TABLE 7: *four-star foods* ****

TYPE OF FOOD	EXAMPLES
Beans, easy to digest (i.e., beans containing fluids)	adzuki sprouts, mung beans
Coconut, green	fresh green coconut meat
Flowers, edible	chrysanthemum, nasturtium, rose, tiger lily
Fruits, succulent (ripe, organic, high energy)	citrus, kiwi, melons, nectarines, peaches, plums, pomegranates
Olives, ripe (unprocessed)	—
Sprouts (light by weight) and green sprouts	alfalfa, broccoli, chia, clover, garlic, onion, radish

from the sun. It is collected by plants in the form of ultraviolet rays, which is energy. The ratings of the listed foods are based on the radiance they contain and emit. Higher levels of food have greater radiance, because their cells are capable of capturing and maintaining greater amounts of the ultraviolet rays of the sun.

Five-star foods (*****) indicate those with the greatest nutritional and electrical frequency available; fewer stars indicate diminished potencies and vitality. Nutritional quality and quantity are created within each plant and are determined by the amount of sun energy contained within the cell structure of the plant.

Please note that even at the lowest levels, cooked food is not mentioned because none of it registers any measurable frequency. Our research shows that cooked vegetables neither contain nor emit energy. Although dairy foods and meat do not contain radiance, both do absorb energy from the body when they are consumed. While cooked food does not contribute energy to your body, dairy and meat are even worse: they deplete your energy reserves.

The lesson to be learned from these observations is basic common sense. Those who consume the least amount of meat have the fewest incidences of man-made disease and illness, while those who consume the highest amount of meat have the most health problems. Those who consume absolutely no animal products have the fewest diseases and health problems.

TABLE 8: *three-star foods* ***

TYPE OF FOOD	EXAMPLES
Fruits, vine grown	currants, grapes, tomatoes
Grains (sprouted, with two-day germination)	all grains
Nuts	all except cashews and peanuts
Sauerkraut	green, purple, and red cabbage
Seeds (sprouted)	flax, hemp, pumpkin, sesame, sunflower
Vegetables (green, yellow, orange, purple, white, and red)	beets, broccoli, brussels sprouts, cabbage (green, red), carrots, cauliflower, celery, corn, cucumber, garlic, lettuce (iceberg), onions (unsprouted), peas, peppers (orange, red), squash (winter), squash (yellow), string beans, sweet potatoes, yams
Vegetables, dehydrated	chives, garlic, green herbal seasonings (organic), onions, peppers (sweet)
Vegetables, green leafy	organic, farm-grown vegetables shipped within forty-eight hours of harvesting and eaten within two weeks after that

Argentineans, Australians, Northern Europeans, and North Americans, the heaviest consumers of animal-based food, are also the sickest based on World Health Organization statistics on cancer, heart disease, and the other maladies of the industrialized world. Ironically, these people are also among the most economically prosperous. Sadly, many of those who are neither prosperous nor carnivorous suffer at the other end of the dietary spectrum as the victims of malnutrition and starvation. As with all areas of life, what is needed is balance: Those with the means must improve their diets; those without the means must be accommodated with health-promoting food.

Using the stars, you can determine what level of energy you would like to achieve. At times, one-star foods are acceptable even for people in the platinum range. The lower energy content of sprouted grain and bean preparations decelerates the metabolism, allowing

TABLE 9: *two-star foods* **

TYPE OF FOOD	EXAMPLES
Beans (sprouted)	all varieties except soy and black
Fruit (grown in northern latitudes)	apples (most), blackberries, blueberries, cherries, cranberries, gooseberries, pears (most), raspberries
Mushrooms (eaten raw)	maitake, reishi, shiitake
Root vegetables	burdock, celery, jicama, parsnip, radish, rutabaga, turnip, yucca
Whole grain preparations (raw, dehydrated living food)	bread, cereal, chips, cookies, pizza crust

healthy weight gain in those who do no resistance exercise. People who are in the bronze or copper realms can use the four- and five-star foods to increase stamina and clarity.

Do not limit yourself or try to maintain unrealistic goals. After reading this chapter, many robust dreamers will say that they want to live exclusively on five-star foods and remain permanently on the platinum platform. When they fail to achieve this objective, they may

TABLE 10: *one-star foods* *

TYPE OF FOOD	EXAMPLES
Chestnuts, raw	—
Grain preparations, dehydrated (stored for more than thirty days)	breads, cereals
Legumes, dehydrated	all beans except soy and black
Nuts and seeds, dehydrated	almonds, Brazil nuts, flax, hazelnuts, hemp, pecans, pine nuts, pistachios (unprocessed), pumpkin, sesame, sunflower, walnuts
Root vegetables, dehydrated	beets, carrots, jicama, sweet potatoes, yams
Salad dressings, raw vegan (prepared in a blender)	all except vinegar-and-oil dressings

relinquish their hopes and sabotage their own dreams. Refined emotions, a positive self-image, constructive experience, and common sense should govern your choices.

If you never fail to do your best, you will progress securely and eventually live in a comfort zone that fits you and your life at that time. However, just because the given level is comfortable, do not get so complacent with it that you fail to constantly try to achieve higher levels of functioning or remain at the highest level once you have reached it. If you are already at the highest level, reside there with the highest level of dignity as well.

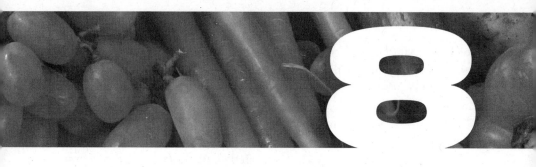

create your own
health support system

Nothing can bring you peace except yourself.

RALPH WALDO EMERSON

Many of you may believe that you are not yet prepared to relinquish your addictions in order to embrace the Hippocrates Lifeforce Program. If you are one of these people, ask yourself the following questions: Am I willing to sacrifice my long-term health to protect a single one of my toxic lifestyle habits? Am I willing to die prematurely in return for holding on to my food addictions?

If you answered no to either or both of these questions, then you may be more ready than you realize to make some dramatic, positive changes in your life. Creating your own support system for participating in the Lifeforce Program involves integrating a practical working knowledge of lifeforce techniques with a psychological framework of inner discipline and an outer network of supportive friends and family. Once you take that important first step, this could become your survival manual for the twenty-first century!

As you know by now, a central theme of this book concerns the need to harness your mind and your beliefs to maintain good health or reclaim a state of wellness. If you cannot summon the self-discipline and commitment to adhere to the Lifeforce Program, then all of the practical strategies and techniques for implementing the program will amount to nothing more than an exercise in futility.

For decades, the most widely implemented self-help regimen on the planet for breaking addictions has been the twelve-step program of Alcoholics Anonymous (AA). These steps have been applied to many other addictive behaviors, from drugs and gambling to pornography and overspending. Harmful food habits and food addictions can be just as dysfunctional and toxic to our well-being as any other addictive behavior, so there is no reason why we cannot apply the same twelve-step principles to breaking the grip these negative patterns have on us.

You can change any of your lifestyle addictions using this simple formula. In the text that follows, you'll find the twelve steps with the wording slightly altered to reflect our emphasis on breaking food addictions. In AA, the reference to God can mean any form of higher power, even the higher power within ourselves. Use "God" or "Higher Power," whichever you feel is more in alignment with your spiritual beliefs.

If we only think of food as a fun or sensory experience designed merely to satisfy our hunger and our taste cravings, we lose sight of food's

the twelve-step program for breaking food addictions

1. We admit that we are powerless in the face of our food addictions—that our life has become unhealthy and unmanageable as a result, and we must make a change.

2. We choose to believe that a Power greater than ourselves can help to restore our health and our ability to manage and control our food addictions.

3. We make a decision to turn our will and our trust over to the care of this Higher Power as we understand it.

4. We agree to undertake a searching and fearless moral inventory of the truth about ourselves in relation to our food dependencies and beliefs.

5. We confess to the Higher Power, to ourselves, and to another human being the exact nature of our cravings and weaknesses.

6. We are entirely ready to remove all of these defects from our lives.

7. We humbly ask the Higher Power to help us to remove our shortcomings.

8. We have made a list of all persons we have harmed as a result of our weakness, and we are willing to make amends to them all, including ourselves.

9. We have made direct amends to such people wherever possible, except when to do so would injure them or others.

10. We continue to take a personal inventory, and when we are weak or wrong will promptly admit it and seek the support of others.

11. We seek through prayer and meditation to improve our conscious contact with God as we understand God or a Higher Power, and we seek to tap into our own power to carry out our desire to control our compulsions.

12. Having had a spiritual awakening or a more enlightened world view as the result of undertaking these steps, we try to carry this message to others and to practice these principles in all our ways of being, both with ourselves and others.

most important purpose and role in life—to provide fuel and medicine for the human body. We know that our harmful attitudes and behaviors regarding food and eating can be reprogrammed. We also realize that it is a serious mistake to wait for a health crisis to jolt us into that awareness or to force us to turn food consumption into a wellness strategy.

If we lack willpower, we can use the twelve-step program to help us break addictive patterns and to set in motion our emotional and spiritual transformation in relationship to our eating, health, and healing. If we allow our addictions to keep seducing us back to the old patterns and habits, we will find the living food lifestyle path to be a difficult and daunting challenge. We just need to flip the channel of our life to a program that benefits our health. It is called the survival channel, and the tuner is in our hands!

eating in the "real" world

When I began this lifestyle in the early 1970s, long before I became director of the Hippocrates Health Institute, it was a period I like to call "the dark ages," a time when public awareness about the benefits of the living food lifestyle—

a lifestyle commitment to healing

At the age of thirty-one, I went into the hospital for what was supposed to be a simple procedure to remove a blood clot on my uterus. However, it turned out to be a grapefruit-sized tumor growing out of my uterus, and it was touching my ovary, bladder, colon, and abdominal wall.

My surgeons removed my uterus and one ovary, and I'm told they did their best to scrape any remaining cells from the various places where the tumor had been touching. The diagnosis was a pelvic sarcoma with a very aggressive cell type. Since it is an uncommon tumor, it is hard to give an accurate statistical prognosis. However, I do know that things were looking grim.

My oncologist, with whom I have a wonderful relationship, gave me six cycles of intensive chemotherapy over the next four months. Four weeks after I completed my conventional therapy, I went into the Hippocrates Lifeforce Program. I was bald, skinny, weak, menopausal, anemic, and had a low white blood cell count. I spent three weeks at Hippocrates, and a different member of my immediate family stayed with me each week. I had a wonderful experience there and took the program home with me (as did each member of my family, much to their surprise!).

I have been juicing five times a day (two wheatgrass, one cucumber, and two green drinks) ever since then and eat the mostly raw, vegan, organic diet I learned about at Hippocrates. I bought a second Champion juicer, which I keep at work so I can juice there. I purchased a sturdy suitcase that allows me to pack a juicer and juicing supplies when I travel. I hired someone to come to my home a few hours a week to help with my food preparation, so that each morning I can put my containers of salad and juice prep in a bag and go to work.

This lifestyle definitely requires a strong commitment, and three years later I am still refining my routine so that it fits more easily into my day. I can assure you that the benefits have been stupendous. I feel well and am told I look well. As best as modern medicine can tell, there is no evidence of cancer in my body.

I became engaged to a wonderful man, and though he eats a fairly standard American diet, he is very supportive and encouraging of what I do.

The best news of all is that my remaining ovary started functioning again. With the support of this lifestyle, I am looking forward to a long life of good times and challenges.

LILLI B. LINK
NEW YORK CITY

both to society and to personal health—was still in its infancy. Once I gave up eating meat, I never touched it again. But it took me another three years to become brave enough to relinquish dairy and my favorite taste sensation of all, ice cream. I was about twenty-three years old, and my decision was made in the face of tremendous peer group pressure, social resistance, and overall ignorance about the nutritional benefits of the lifestyle, much less the ethical implications.

So-called nutritional experts warned me that I would destroy my health by adopting a living food diet, but I lost one hundred pounds of excess body weight and became not only healthier but kinder to myself and others. I had slipped into eating raw food one summer while living in Oregon, and then I read Ann Wigmore's book. That really opened my eyes to the potential advantages of this lifestyle. I paid a visit to Hippocrates, which was then located in Boston, and was invited to join the staff. Most of the guests at that time had chronic or catastrophic illnesses, and as I watched these people recover using the living food diet, I felt as though I was in the presence of God. It became absolutely clear to me that the Hippocrates Program and lifestyle were tools to open the hearts and minds of people and enable them to lead happier and more productive lives.

To succeed on this diet for the long-term, we must adapt our way of life, depending upon the environment in which we live. To be alone and isolated while trying to succeed with this lifestyle is much more difficult than if you create your own support system with family or friends or seek out like-minded people in the community. If you are personally committed to a lifestyle of integrity, you will attract people who will provide both practical and emotional support.

Trying to embrace this lifestyle just halfway using moderation may pose more challenges for you than if you were to go "cold turkey" and proceed all of the way at once. T. Colin Campbell described the dangers of moderation this way in *The China Study*: "There are three excellent reasons to go all the way. First, following this diet requires a radical shift in your thinking about food. It's more work to just do it halfway. If you plan for animal-based products, you'll eat them—and you'll almost certainly eat more than you should. Second, you'll feel deprived. Instead of viewing your new food habit as being able to eat all the plant-based food you want, you'll be seeing it in terms of having to limit yourself, which is not conducive to staying on the diet long term. If you had friends who had been smokers all of their lives and looked to you for advice, would you tell them to cut down to only two cigarettes a day, or would you tell them to quit smoking altogether? It's in this way that I'm telling you that moderation, even with the best of intentions, sometimes makes it more difficult to succeed."

The Internet has opened up an entire world of new opportunities for exploring, establishing, and reinforcing this lifestyle. There are vegan romance Web sites where you can find like-minded mates. There are living food chat rooms where practical tips and inspirational stories about this lifestyle are exchanged. There are living food trips and cruises available. There are a multitude of resources just a Google away from your fingertips. We are in the midst of a true renaissance when it comes to this lifestyle, and our choices are only limited by our imaginations and our willingness to be resourceful.

Naturally, everyone has questions or concerns about how to live this life and do so while swimming against the strong prevailing currents of modern culture. My first caution is to examine your questions carefully. Are they truly just innocent questions, or do your fears and self-sabotaging behaviors masquerade as legitimate queries? Are your questions simply rationalizations designed to undermine your commitment?

Here are three of the most commonly asked questions about the raw food diet:

1. How do I persuade my family to adopt the lifestyle?

The most effective way to teach other people, especially your friends and family, about the living food lifestyle is simply to live it! When you make changes in your life that maximize your health, other people will learn from your example, because they will see firsthand how healthy and vibrant you have become.

In addition to setting an example, there are a series of actions that you will need to take to protect yourself and those you love. First, remove the most dangerous foods from your kitchen, including foods that contains excess fat, protein, sugar, salt, and chemical additives. Also eliminate alcohol and vinegar. Replace what you remove with nutritious fare as you wean your family from their dependence on toxins. Rather than making your loved ones feel deprived, simply introduce them to more healthful alternatives. Replace refined grain products with whole grains. Replace conventional dairy products with low-fat goat, almond, rice, and soy varieties. Replace white potatoes with yams and sweet potatoes. Replace sugar-filled desserts with fresh fruit cocktails or banana ice cream made with fresh bananas.

Next, replace hazardous methods of cooking, such as microwaving and frying, with baking, dehydrating, and steaming. Make the centerpiece of every meal a mixed salad of sprouts and various in-season vegetables, especially the green leafy ones. Experiment by making salad dressings and sauces that rely on avocados, soaked nuts, or soaked beans as their base. Finally, prepare at least one recipe from any good vegan or vegetarian cookbook with every meal until this becomes a custom within your family.

2. What preparations should I make when traveling?

Use the Internet to contact natural food stores or vegetarian restaurants in your destination city, or search for a variety of organic foods sold at farmers markets by organic growers. Many restaurants now have salad bars, but the obvious question to raise with restaurant employees is whether the produce is organically grown.

Planning what to eat on long plane trips requires some advance thought and maybe a few inquiries. Contact the airline to see if it offers vegetarian or vegan meals, and if so, reserve one for yourself. If it does not, prepare your own meal package with sprouts, spelt bread, and dehydrated snacks. Carry an ample supply of distilled water. Airlines such as Swiss Air and Lufthansa serve organic food on request. Most cruise lines do as well.

a lifestyle that keeps health issues at bay

Prior to nine years ago, sadly, my diet was the Standard American Diet—SAD. It consisted of heavy meat and dairy consumption featuring steak and potatoes, cheeses, pepperoni pizza, pasta with meatballs, bread and more bread. I also led a life of health challenges.

At the age of six I almost died from an infection in my heart. This was due to mitral valve prolapse, a faulty heart valve, which allowed contaminated blood to enter my heart. I was given megadoses of antibiotics for six months and recovered, but I was left with permanent heart damage to the electrical muscle. My entire life I have had tachycardia (rapid heart action), a heart murmur, angina, and an irregular heartbeat. Due to the overuse of antibiotics, my immune system was severely compromised, and I was constantly sick after that with pneumonia, bronchitis, tonsillitis, flus, and colds.

When I turned sixteen, I got tonsillitis again. This time I did not respond to antibiotics, and I developed a fever of 105 degrees F and lost fourteen pounds in three days; I was dying for the second time. They rushed me into surgery because my tonsils were so enlarged they had almost closed off my windpipe. The surgery was catastrophic, and I lost part of my throat muscle tissue.

Then at eighteen, I got mononucleosis. At about twenty years of age, it was discovered that I had polycystic ovary disease, which gave me multiple and debilitating menstrual symptoms, including severe pain and weakness and flulike symptoms. Over the next decade, I developed multiple inhalant and food allergies, systemic *Candida*, multiple chemical sensitivities, and chronic fatigue syndrome.

The final straw was when I reached my mid-thirties and contracted Lyme disease, though I still had all the other issues—head-to-toe aches and pains, fatigue, and poor complexion. I was also overweight and had no strength. This was the third time I almost died. I was so sick I couldn't work for a month and had to take a leave of absence from my job. The Lyme disease degenerated three of my joints, the most severe being my left shoulder, and I could not use my left arm for nearly three years.

At this point I was ready to try something new—for thirty years I had done everything the doctors told me, took every drug, and had a few surgeries—and I never did get better. I started to read books on health, and most emphasized diet and lifestyle. I initially stopped going to doctors, taking medications, and having procedures done. I started to eat all-vegetarian meals at thirty-nine years of age, and six months later, I became a vegan.

I gave up meat, literally overnight, but cheese was more difficult. I felt best when I was vegan. In my home and at work I am vegan. When I go out, I stick to vegetarianism (no animal flesh in nine years—no beef, chicken, or fish). I find that the longer I live this lifestyle, the easier it is to maintain it. My cravings have changed over the years, and I now enjoy foods today that I did not a year ago.

My shoulder completely healed within six months of becoming a vegan. Now, as long as I remain vegan, I have no joint symptoms, but when I stray from the diet, I get a very rapid reminder of my joint issues. Presently, I have a great complexion, abundant energy, no pain, and no chronic fatigue, and I test negative for Epstein-Barr virus, Lyme disease, and *Candida*. And I have an exhilaration about life that is mirrored by my physical stamina.

The process of changing our lives begins with our thoughts. The trick for success in the Lifeforce Program is to engage in active, positive decision making, free of any habituated impulses. Will this be difficult? Perhaps at first, depending on your history of dependence on toxic food and your level of commitment to your goals. After that, then the program just becomes a part of your normal life.

J. MICHELE VILLAREALE
WEST PALM BEACH, FLORIDA

When you are dining out, remember that many Japanese, Chinese, Middle Eastern, Greek, and northern Italian restaurants offer choices of nutritious vegetable dishes, though most conventional American and European restaurants do not. In many major cities of the world, chestnuts are available as a filling and nutritious snack; they are sold by vendors on the streets of Paris, New York, and elsewhere.

Being resourceful with this lifestyle will eventually become second nature. When my wife, Anna Maria, and I traveled to Russia, for instance, we knew we would not be able to purchase organic vegetables very easily in that country. So we brought two large suitcases of our preferred foods with us. I even take sprouts with me in my briefcase when I travel to business meetings. You might try arranging in advance to have organic foods shipped to your destination when you travel. In Europe there are services that supply organic produce that has been picked no more than five days prior to delivery.

3. Will raw food deplete my physical stamina?

For a clear and convincing answer to this question, consider the experience of Doug Walsh, a Colorado raw food vegan since 1996, who demonstrated how the human body thrives on a raw food diet by hiking three thousand miles from Mexico to Canada along the Conti-

five years on the living food diet

Before I discovered this lifestyle, I was eating a diet that included meat and dairy, and I gained twenty pounds of extra weight since beginning college. After graduating from the University of Kansas, I discovered I had a new passion for living a natural lifestyle. I immediately transitioned to a vegan diet, but that diet consisted of mostly junk food, even though it was vegan. I was eating frozen burritos, pasta, and lots of fruit. It wasn't until I picked up *The Raw Life* by Paul Nison that I began to discover the power of eating a living food diet.

I began to regularly frequent the health food store by my house and developed friendships with other people interested in this lifestyle. It was fun spending lunch at the juice bar, eating salads and connecting with other like-minded people. The most difficult part of transitioning to this diet was socializing with my friends and family who were not familiar with this way of eating. I seemed to always attract attention when I would attend any social gathering, because I wasn't eating the sweet desserts and other food that would be provided. I learned to not say much about what I could eat, but if someone inquired about it, I had no problem answering. I actually loved to talk about my new lifestyle and way of eating! But I learned fast that people are more receptive if you don't preach to them, and the people who are interested will ask you questions.

nental Divide Trail. It was Earth Day, April 22, 2005, and Walsh set out under cosponsorship of the Hippocrates Health Institute, hiking an average of a marathon a day, every day for the entire five months it took him to make the arduous journey. This "Lance Armstrong of raw food," as we call him, later described his feat to us this way:

"I became a vegan in 1988 after reading *Diet for a New America* by John Robbins. It was a natural progression for me. I have always been interested in health because I love the outdoors. I realize that I must be healthy to be able to do what I love, which is to play outside! Over the years, my vegan diet was refined, and I became healthier and healthier. Two influential books that led me to living food were *Conscious Eating* by Gabriel Cousens and the Diamonds' *Fit For Life*. It made total sense to me. Eating food that is still full of the energy from the earth was the obvious way to go. That energy is channeled to me,

Committing to this lifestyle has been an exciting roller-coaster ride for me. It has been a process with ups and downs. It is so exciting to discover new information. It's like unpeeling layers of truth that were unavailable to me in the past. I learn something new, and I adjust my lifestyle and diet accordingly to see how I feel. It's amazing how my body has changed and healed from years of overeating and substance abuse. My mind is incredibly clear. One of my favorite improvements is the quality of sleep I have and the clarity of my dreams. I have increased energy and stamina, and I have so much freedom now that I am not addicted to caffeine and other harmful substances.

My ability to maintain this lifestyle becomes easier every day. Once you commit to improving your health and life, your determination will empower you to make the correct choices concerning your diet and lifestyle. Staying focused on a goal and surrounding yourself with like-minded individuals are important factors in maintaining this way of life. I try not to be too hard on myself and to set realistic goals that I can meet. I learned that I am always changing, and how I approach this way of living is always changing. Discovering the living food lifestyle has been the greatest gift and has changed my life in ways I never imagined.

ANDREA NISON
WEST PALM BEACH, FLORIDA

and I get so excited about life. I love this lifestyle. You don't have to deprive yourself or make sacrifices to be healthy.

"It was the longest hike I have ever done, somewhere between 3,000 and 3,200 miles. The elevation of this hike was continuously high, averaging over eleven thousand feet. Walking a marathon or more per day at that elevation is definitely a challenge, even for a raw foodist. The weather conditions were brutal at times, and we were constantly exposed to rain, snow, wind, hail, and thunderstorms with dangerous lightning. You name it, we got it on this trail.

"I hiked with a friend of mine, Eric, basically the whole way. He is not a raw food person. He's not even a vegetarian. However, after hiking with me, he wants to become a raw foodist because he saw the obvious advantages of my lifestyle. Eric is fourteen years younger than I am but suffered much more than I did on this hike. He also had much less stamina that I had."

embracing the new you

You have now come to the end of the beginning—the beginning of your whole life, nourished by living food, free of toxins, fully functional, and fulfilled. And all that you have to do to continue is what you have been doing since you started reading this book. But be wary and watchful of falling back into the self-destructive patterns that led you to this book in the first place. To paraphrase former baseball great Satchel Page, if you do not fall back, the past cannot control you.

Soon after I became director of the Hippocrates Health Institute in 1981, we sent out a survey to about eighteen thousand graduates of the Lifeforce Program asking if they were still following the program, and if so, to what extent. More than half the addresses were no longer valid, but we still got nearly three thousand answers from the mailing. We found that 47 percent of the respondents were still following the program. Six percent had gone bonkers and were eating fried chicken and hamburgers. The rest were either vegetarian or vegan, or aspiring to be most of the time.

To have that many people continue on a program so at odds with our prevailing culture is really quite an extraordinary commentary on both the quality of our program and the human desire for health and wellness. We continue to conduct periodic smaller surveys, because

80 percent of our guests return to our on-site program for tune-ups. Some of them come back because they have gone off the program and need to reexperience the structure that we provide. But on average, we still find that half of our graduates stick with the program. (We use the word "guests" rather than "clients" or "patients" because we want everyone to feel equal and responsible in the process of addressing his or her own health challenges.)

Everything that you continue to learn from this book will mean nothing unless you apply it every day in every way. Like all practical learning, the guidelines that constitute this book must be practiced and lived in order for them to be effective. In living the program, you will need to live your best; and in living your best, you will be your best and give your best to the world around you.

And so, like the great circle of life, we have returned to the beginning, to each individual's responsibility for the totality of his or her own health and well-being. If we think of all of life—now and forever—as the universal totality that it is, how can harming any life not be harmful to all of life? As Dag Hammarskjöld, the late secretary general of the United Nations, advised us, "Our work for peace must begin within the private world of each of us."

From each of those worlds—individually and together—we must apply the Golden Rule and the basic principle of the Hippocratic oath, "First, do no harm," to each thought, each movement, and each action. We must do so until the Golden Rule and that principle flow from person to person, from people to other creatures, from other creatures to nature, from nature back to people and other creatures, from place to place, from age to age, until the entirety of the planet is enveloped in a cocoon of love, goodness, and eternal bliss.

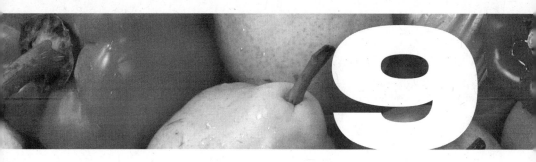

special recipes from the Hippocrates kitchen

You will find literally thousands of raw vegan recipes online and in books that support the Hippocrates nutrition program. One of my favorites from among these books is *Healthful Cuisine: Over 150 Raw Vegan Recipes*, written by my wife, Anna Maria Clement, and Chef Kelly Serbonich. Their book not only features great cuisine, it educates readers on the basics of soaking and sprouting, juicing and blending, and mastering the process of food dehydration.

The following recipes, all used at the Hippocrates Health Institute by our chefs, will give you a sampling of the vast variety of tasty foods that are also nutritious, health promoting, and healing.

color-me-cauliflower salad

Yield: 2 to 4 servings

This tasty salad works well for any occasion.

½ head cauliflower, cut into bite-size pieces

½ head broccoli, cut into bite-size pieces

2 red bell peppers, chopped

½ cup minced fresh parsley

1 cup raw pine nuts, soaked 12 hours

¼ cup water

½ teaspoon ground ginger

2 tablespoons Bragg Liquid Aminos

1 garlic clove, chopped

To make the salad, combine the cauliflower and broccoli in a mixing bowl. Add the bell peppers and parsley and toss gently.

To make the dressing, drain and rinse the pine nuts. Transfer them to a blender along with the water and ginger, and process until smooth. Stir in the Bragg Liquid Aminos and garlic. Pour over the vegetables and toss gently. Let rest for 30 minutes at room temperature before serving to allow the flavors to blend.

VARIATIONS

- Add grated fresh ginger and Italian seasoning to taste.
- Omit the Bragg Liquid Aminos and add kelp powder or dulse granules to taste.

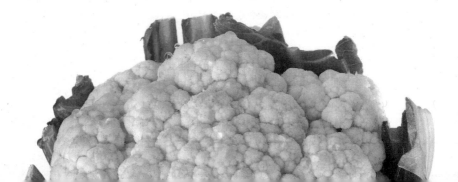

hummus-a-tune

This is a great dip that can be eaten with raw flax crackers or your favorite raw veggies.

2 cups chickpeas, soaked 12 hours and sprouted 24 hours

½ cup water

2 to 4 garlic cloves, chopped

1½ teaspoons ground cumin (optional)

¼ cup freshly squeezed lemon juice

3 tablespoons raw tahini

3 tablespoons Bragg Liquid Aminos

ombine the chickpeas, water, and garlic in a blender, and process into a smooth paste. Add the cumin, if using, lemon juice, tahini, and Bragg Liquid Aminos, and process until well combined. Let rest for 30 minutes at room temperature before serving.

VARIATIONS

- Stir ¼ bunch chopped parsley into the blended mixture.
- Omit the Bragg Liquid Aminos and add kelp powder or dulse granules to taste.

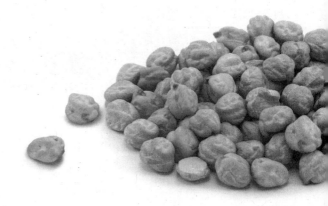

basic guacamole

Yield: 4 to 6 servings

This tasty dip can be eaten on its own or with raw flax crackers, carrots, or other favorite vegetables for dipping.

4 large avocados, diced

½ bunch cilantro, basil, or dill, chopped

½ cup sliced scallions

1 small red bell pepper, diced

2 garlic cloves, chopped

Freshly squeezed lemon juice

Cayenne

Combine the avocados, cilantro, scallions, bell pepper, and garlic in a mixing bowl or food processor, and blend just until well combined but still chunky. Season with lemon juice and cayenne to taste.

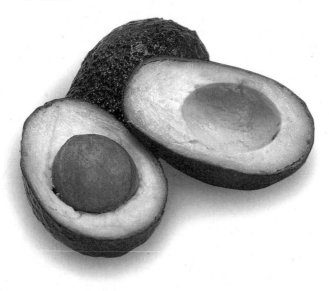

foreign fantasy

This salad makes a nutritious addition to any meal.

½ cup raw hazelnuts or almonds, soaked 12 hours

2 cups sliced red or green cabbage

½ cup julienne jicama or sliced fresh water chestnuts

½ cup fresh green peas

½ cup dulse, soaked

1 red bell pepper, chopped

1 cup water

2 tablespoons flaxseeds

1 cup sliced red bell peppers

To make the salad, drain and rinse the hazelnuts and transfer them to a mixing bowl. Add the cabbage, jicama, peas, and dulse, and toss until well combined.

To make the dressing, combine the chopped bell pepper, water, and flaxseeds in a blender, and process until smooth. Pour over the salad and garnish with the sliced bell pepper. Let rest in the refrigerator for 15 to 30 minutes before serving.

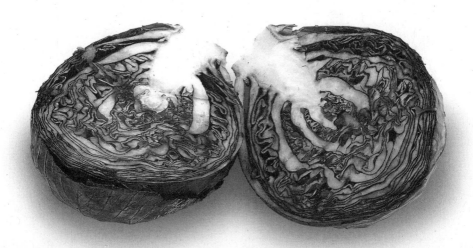

sesame-mushroom medley

Yield: 2 to 3 servings

This salad's flavor and texture get even better after it marinates.

1 pound shiitake mushrooms, sliced

1 red bell pepper, diced

Scallions, diagonally sliced

2 limes, juiced

¼ cup raw sesame seeds

1 tablespoon cold-pressed olive oil or organic sesame oil

1 teaspoon ground coriander

Pinch of cayenne

Bragg Liquid Aminos

Combine the mushrooms, bell pepper, and scallions to taste in a large mixing bowl. Add the lime juice, sesame seeds, olive oil, coriander, and cayenne and toss gently. Season with Bragg Liquid Aminos to taste.

VARIATION

• Add finely minced or pressed fresh garlic and ginger to taste.

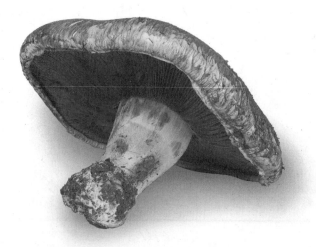

kale and mustard

Here's a salad with a spicy kick. It provides a zesty way to add dark leafy greens to your diet.

    2 to 3 bunches kale

    2 large red bell peppers, sliced

    3 to 4 dehydrated nut or seed patties (optional)

    2 tablespoons dry mustard

    4 tablespoons freshly squeezed lemon juice

    Cold-pressed olive oil, as needed

To make the salad, remove and discard the kale stems and tear the leaves into bite-size pieces. Place in a bowl with the bell peppers and optional patties.

To make the dressing, combine the dry mustard with just enough water to make a paste. Add the lemon juice and as much olive oil as necessary to achieve the desired consistency. Pour over the vegetables and toss gently. Let marinate at room temperature for 1 hour before serving.

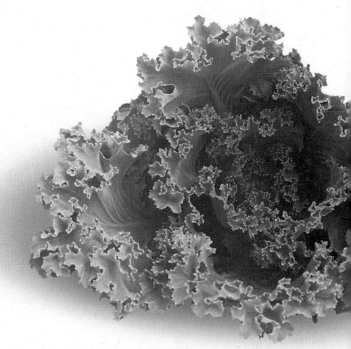

squash and potatoes

Yield: 4 to 6 servings

This salad adds variety to your diet and is a healthful alternative to potato salad.

3 cups cubed yellow squash

3 cups cubed zucchini

1 cup grated sweet potatoes

1 cup grated carrots

¼ cup chopped fresh tarragon

3 garlic cloves, crushed

3 tablespoons cold-pressed olive oil or flaxseed oil

Bragg Liquid Aminos

Combine the yellow squash and zucchini in a large bowl. Add the sweet potatoes, carrots, tarragon, and garlic. Add the oil, and toss until all the ingredients are evenly distributed. Season with Bragg Liquid Aminos to taste.

VARIATION

* Omit the Bragg Liquid Aminos and add kelp powder or dulse granules to taste.

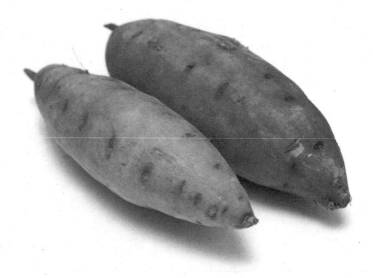

mixed sea vegetable salad

A delicious Asian treat, this salad is highly nutritious.

1 ounce dulse, sliced

1 ounce arame

1 ounce hijiki

2 nori sheets

1 cup shredded carrots

1 cup shredded daikon

6 scallions, diagonally sliced

2 large lemons, juiced

3 tablespoons raw sesame seeds

Bragg Liquid Aminos

Soak the dulse, arame, and hijiki separately until softened. Rinse all three separately and drain. Cut the nori into 1-inch squares. Combine the dulse, arame, hijiki, and nori in a large bowl. Add the carrots, daikon, and scallions. Sprinkle the lemon juice and sesame seeds over the salad and mix well. Season with Bragg Liquid Aminos to taste.

VARIATION

- For an Asian flavor, add grated fresh ginger to taste.

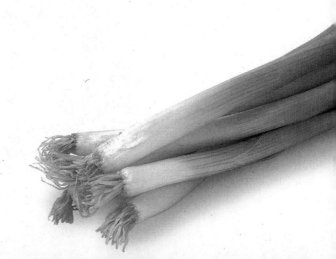

bean-artichoke medley

Try this salad for a classic Italian dining experience.

2 cups sliced wax beans

1 head radicchio, coarsely chopped

1 head endive, coarsely chopped

½ cup pitted black olives, sliced in half

1 cup raw artichoke hearts

3 tablespoons cold-pressed olive oil

Herbal seasoning

Combine the wax beans, radicchio, and endive in a large bowl and mix well. Add the olives and artichoke hearts, and toss until well combined. Pour the olive oil over the mixture, and add herbal seasoning to taste. Toss until everything is evenly distributed.

VARIATION

- Add freshly squeezed lemon juice to taste.

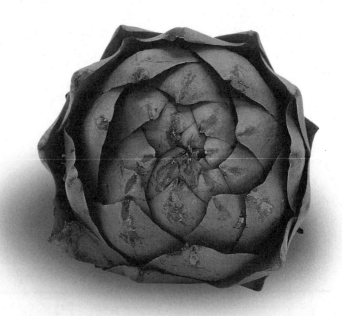

wasabi bok choy

This exotic salad is delicious, but be careful with the wasabi. It is hot and spicy, so use it sparingly.

2 pounds bok choy

Wasabi powder

1 medium, sweet onion, thinly sliced

8 ounces bean sprouts

Wash the bok choy and slice it into bite-size pieces. Transfer the slightly damp bok choy to a mixing bowl, and sprinkle the wasabi powder over it to taste. Add the onion and bean sprouts. Toss gently and serve.

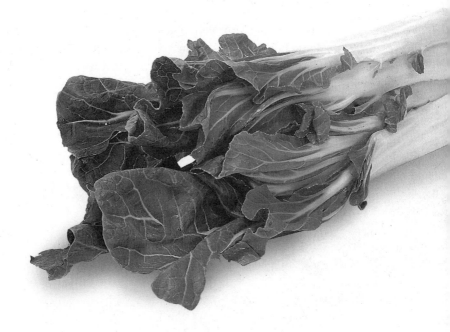

Italian vegetable medley

Yield: 4 to 6 servings

Here's a traditional dish that is delightful to eat and easy to prepare.

½ pound zucchini, sliced

½ pound yellow squash, sliced

½ pound red bell pepper, sliced

½ pound broccoli florets, sliced

1 head radicchio, shredded (optional)

¼ cup chopped fresh basil

¼ cup cold-pressed olive oil

¼ cup freshly squeezed lemon juice

2 to 3 garlic cloves, minced

3 tablespoons pizza seasoning (optional)

Combine the zucchini, yellow squash, bell pepper, and broccoli in a large bowl and toss gently. Add the optional radicchio and basil and toss again. Add the olive oil, lemon juice, and garlic, and toss until evenly distributed. If desired, sprinkle with pizza seasoning to taste and toss once more. Let marinate for 1 hour before serving.

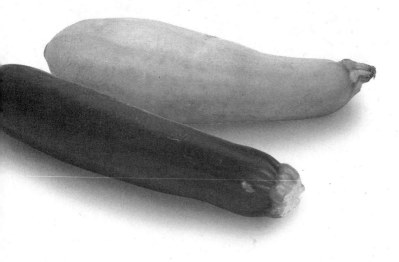

sesame a-mung the broccoli

This is a creamy Asian dish that is light but filling.

2 cups broccoli florets

2 cups mung bean sprouts

1 cup sliced red bell peppers

2 tablespoons raw sesame oil

2 tablespoons Bragg Liquid Aminos

1 tablespoon ground coriander

½ teaspoon cayenne

¼ cup raw sesame seeds, soaked for 2 to 3 hours

To make the salad, combine the broccoli, sprouts, and bell peppers in a medium bowl. To make the dressing, blend or whisk the oil, Bragg Liquid Aminos, coriander, and cayenne until well combined. Pour over the vegetables. Drain and rinse the sesame seeds and add them to the salad. Toss gently. Let rest for 30 minutes before serving.

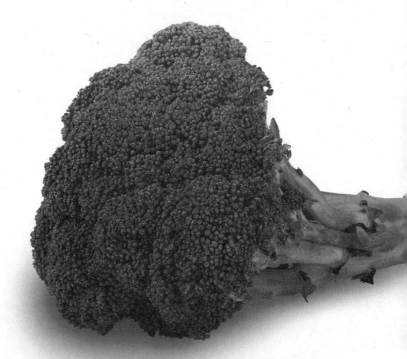

green goddess salad dressing

Yield: 2 to 4 servings

Pour this wonderful taste treat over any vegetable salad.

1 large avocado

1 small onion, quartered

2 celery stalks, cut into 2-inch pieces

¼ cup fresh parsley

¼ cup fresh dill

¼ cup fresh basil

¼ cup watercress

1 cucumber, unpeeled and quartered

1 lemon, juiced

1 garlic clove

Cucumber juice or water, as needed

Bragg Liquid Aminos, kelp powder, or dulse granules

Combine the avocado, onion, and celery in a blender, and process until smooth. Add the parsley, dill, basil, and watercress and process again. Add the cucumber, lemon juice, and garlic. Process until smooth, adding cucumber juice as needed to achieve the desired consistency. Season with Bragg Liquid Aminos to taste.

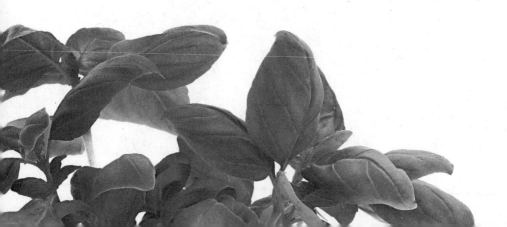

red ranger salad dressing

Yield: 2 to 4 servings

Versatile enough for any vegetable combination, this blended salad dressing will keep in the refrigerator for up to three days.

2 cups raw almonds, soaked 12 hours

1 cup fresh basil

2 garlic cloves

Water, as needed

6 large red bell peppers, sliced

Bragg Liquid Aminos, kelp powder, or dulse granules

Drain and rinse the almonds. Transfer to a blender along with the basil and garlic. Gradually add just enough water to facilitate processing (the mixture should have the consistency of thin pancake batter). With the blender running on medium speed, drop in the bell pepper slices one by one through the cap opening in the lid, and process until completely smooth. Season with Bragg Liquid Aminos to taste.

VARIATION

- Add 3 tablespoons pizza seasoning.

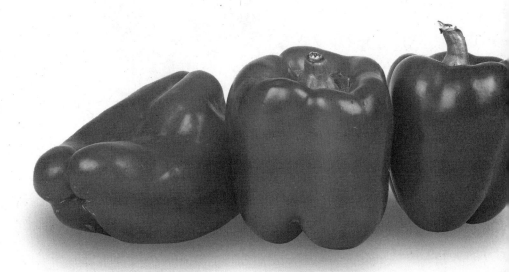

pecan delight salad dressing

Yield: 2 to 4 servings

If you like nutty-tasting salad dressings, this recipe is for you.

2 cups raw pecans, soaked 12 hours

½ cup coarsely chopped fresh parsley

¼ cup sliced red onions

2 to 3 garlic cloves

Cucumber juice or water

Bragg Liquid Aminos

Drain and rinse the pecans. Transfer to a blender along with the parsley, onions, and garlic. Gradually add just enough cucumber juice to facilitate processing; the mixture should be smooth and creamy. Season with Bragg Liquid Aminos to taste.

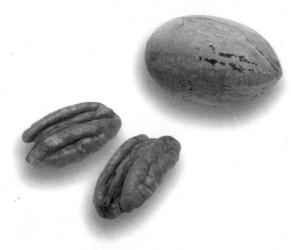

cold asparagus soup

This summertime treat is a meal in itself.

3 cups sliced carrots or, ½ cup fresh carrot juice

2 cups sliced asparagus

¼ cup raw tahini

3 garlic cloves

½ teaspoon grated fresh ginger

Bragg Liquid Aminos, kelp powder, or dulse granules

¼ cup coarsely chopped chives

Combine the carrots, asparagus, tahini, garlic, and ginger in a blender or food processor, and process until smooth. Season with Bragg Liquid Aminos to taste. Chill in the refrigerator for 1 hour. Garnish with the chives just before serving.

VARIATION

- Omit the carrots, tahini, and ginger, and add 1 avocado, cut into chunks, and 2 celery stalks, chopped.

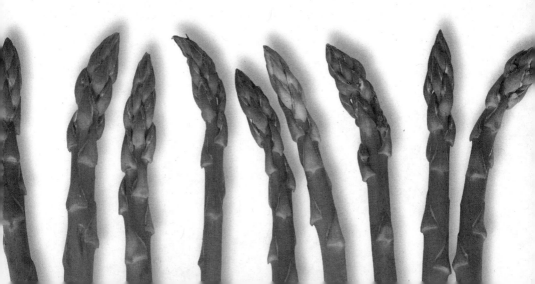

cold carrot-almond soup

Yield: 2 to 3 servings

This is a sweet and satisfying treat that is sure to please your taste buds.

1 cup raw almonds, soaked 12 hours

3 cups fresh carrot juice

1 red or yellow bell pepper, coarsely chopped

1 garlic clove

½ bunch dill, parsley, basil, or cilantro

Bragg Liquid Aminos, kelp powder, or dulse granules

Drain and rinse the almonds. Transfer to a blender along with the carrot juice, bell pepper, and garlic, and process until smooth. Add the dill and process again. Season with Bragg Liquid Aminos to taste.

VARIATION

• Instead of almonds, use ¼ cup raw pine nuts, soaked 12 hours.

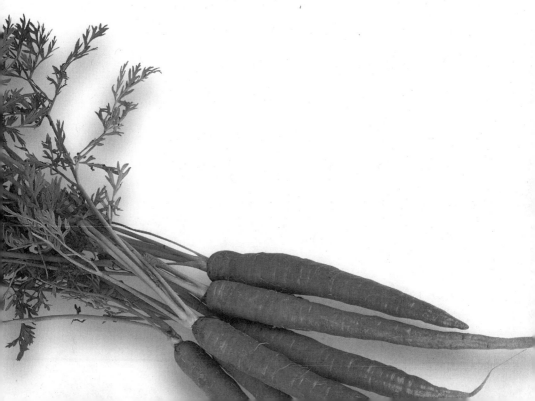

cold avocado-spinach soup

Yield: 2 to 3 servings

Creamy and nutritious, this soup can be a starter or an entire meal.

- 4 cups fresh carrot or cucumber juice
- 2 avocados, coarsely chopped
- 3 garlic cloves
- 1½ pounds spinach, stems removed
- Grated nutmeg
- Bragg Liquid Aminos, kelp powder, or dulse granules

Combine the carrot juice, avocados, and garlic in a blender, and process until smooth. With the blender running on low speed, gradually add the spinach through the cap opening in the lid, and process until evenly incorporated and smooth. Season with nutmeg and Bragg Liquid Aminos to taste.

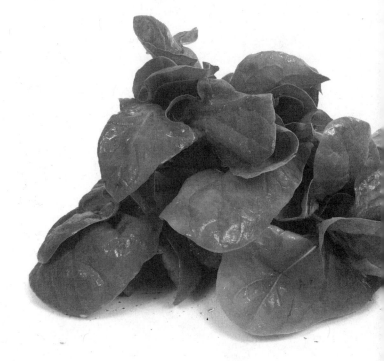

mock tuna salad

This dish offers the texture of tuna without any fishy ingredients.

3 cups raw walnuts, soaked 12 hours

3 cups chopped carrots

1 medium onion, sliced

1 cup chopped celery

½ cup chopped fresh parsley

¼ cup fresh tarragon

¼ cup fresh dill

3 garlic cloves

2 lemons, juiced

2 cups dehydrated vegetables (optional)

Bragg Liquid Aminos, kelp powder, or dulse granules

Fresh greens, for garnish (optional)

Drain and rinse the walnuts. Process the walnuts and carrots through a Champion juicer fitted with the blank screen. Transfer to a mixing bowl. Combine the onion, celery, parsley, tarragon, dill, and garlic in a food processor fitted with the S blade, and pulse until coarsely chopped. Add to the walnut and carrot mixture, and stir until evenly combined. Add the lemon juice and optional dehydrated vegetables and mix again. Season with Bragg Liquid Aminos to taste. Form into the desired shape. Garnish with fresh greens, if desired, and serve.

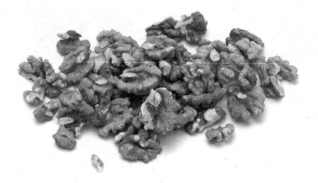

pumpkin and walnut loaf

This dish can be made a day in advance and refrigerated. The resting time will allow the flavors to blend, making it even more delicious.

2 cups raw walnuts, soaked 12 hours

2 cups raw pumpkin seeds, soaked 6 hours

1 cup sliced carrots

1 cup chopped red bell peppers

1 cup diced onions

1 cup chopped fresh parsley

1 cup dehydrated or fresh mushrooms

2 garlic cloves, crushed

2 tablespoons raw tahini (optional)

Fresh herbs, for garnish (optional)

Drain and rinse the walnuts and pumpkin seeds, and process them with the carrots through a Champion juicer fitted with the blank screen. Alternatively, place the walnuts, pumpkin seeds, and carrots in a food processor fitted with the S blade, and process until smooth. Transfer to a large mixing bowl.

Place the bell peppers, onions, parsley, mushrooms, and garlic in a food processor or blender, and pulse until the mixture is well combined but still chunky. Add to the walnut mixture and mix well. Stir in the optional tahini and mix again. Place on a serving dish and form into the desired shape. Garnish with fresh herbs, if desired.

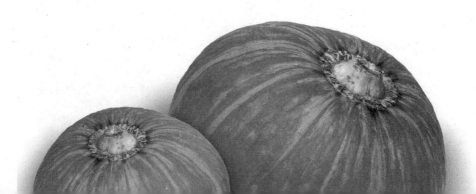

mushroom dip

This special-occasion recipe is versatile enough to satisfy most group events. Serve it with slices of your favorite vegetables or raw flax crackers.

1 cup raw sunflower seeds, soaked 8 to 12 hours

½ cup raw walnuts, soaked 8 to 12 hours

3 cups mushrooms, coarsely chopped

1 carrot, chopped

1 zucchini, chopped

1 red bell pepper, chopped

½ cup chopped scallions

½ celery stalk, chopped

⅓ cup water, plus more as needed

1 tablespoon cold-pressed olive oil

2 teaspoons Bragg Liquid Aminos

Italian seasoning (optional)

Drain and rinse the sunflower seeds and walnuts, and transfer to a food processor fitted with the S blade. Add the mushrooms, carrot, zucchini, bell pepper, scallions, celery, and water, and process until well combined. Add the olive oil and Bragg Liquid Aminos, and process until smooth. Add a small amount of water, if necessary, to facilitate blending and achieve the desired consistency. Stir in Italian seasoning to taste, if desired.

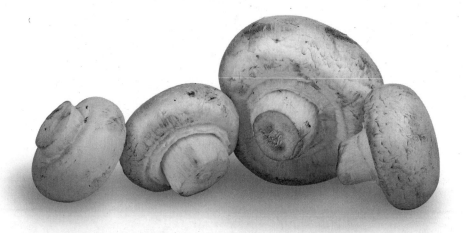

holiday nut loaf

Yield: 4 to 6 servings

This festive treat can be made a day in advance and refrigerated, so you can enjoy the holiday too.

1 cup raw almonds, soaked 8 to 12 hours

½ cup raw sunflower seeds, soaked 8 to 12 hours

½ cup raw sesame seeds, soaked 8 to 12 hours

2 large carrots, sliced or chopped

1 small red bell pepper, sliced or chopped

1 celery stalk, sliced or chopped

¼ cup chopped onions

2 tablespoons chopped fresh parsley

2 garlic cloves

Bragg Liquid Aminos, kelp powder, or dulse granules

Italian seasoning

Drain and rinse the almonds, sunflower seeds, and sesame seeds. Transfer to a food processor fitted with the S blade, and add the carrots, bell pepper, celery, onions, parsley, and garlic. Process until the mixture is well combined and the almonds are thoroughly ground. Season with Bragg Liquid Aminos and Italian seasoning to taste. Form into the desired shape and serve.

VARIATION

- Instead of Italian seasoning, try fresh or dried oregano, basil, thyme, or dill; fresh cilantro; ground cumin; or ground coriander.

NOTE

- Stored in the refrigerator, Holiday Nut Loaf will keep for 2 days.

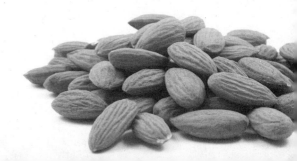

10

therapeutic
juicing

T he nutritional essence of plants is best derived from their juice. Blood is literally the lifeblood that maintains and builds our bodies and juices are its nutritional equivalent. Sunlight infuses all life; plants are the storehouses of nature's captured and distributed sunlight. Juices are among the most important supplemental foods because of the combined potency of nutrition and captured vitality of sunlight they contain.

Condensed nutrition derived from a large quantity of plants provides nourishment that includes vitamins, minerals, trace minerals, oxygen, enzymes, hormones, and phytonutrients. Drink fresh juice within fifteen minutes after it has been extracted to obtain all of its multifaceted nutritional benefits.

The two most common sources of juice are vegetables and fruits. The juice of grasses, sprouts, fresh herbs, and edible flowers can be added to either of these. Research conducted by the Hippocrates Health Institute reveals that disease might result from the consumption of undiluted fruit juices. We encourage the consumption of green vegetable juices and sprout juices and discourage the consumption of fruit juice. A healthy person can consume a combination of approximately

TABLE 11: *therapeutic sprout juices*

SPROUTED SEED JUICE	BENEFITS
Alfalfa	Strengthens blood, which in turn builds strong tissue, reduces edema, and strengthens muscle and bone.
Anise	Good for the respiratory and cardiovascular systems. Also enhances the development of T cells associated with the immune system.
Broccoli	High in phytonutrients. Reduces the potential for mutagenic growths, including cancer. Facilitates healthy and consistent elimination.
Cabbage	Helps to combat an irritated or inflamed digestive tract, ulcers, cancer, osteoarthritis, and osteoporosis.
Cantaloupe	Increases sperm and egg production. Regulates blood sugar, whether low or high.
Cayenne	Countervails heart attack, stroke, and deficient circulation, and benefits those who have had these conditions. Strengthens the cardiovascular and circulatory systems.
Cress	Builds blood by multiplying red blood cells, decreases toxins in the respiratory system, prevents fibroids and cysts, and acts as an anticarcinogen.
Fennel	Builds white and red blood cells. Increases digestive enzymes.
Fenugreek	Fights gastrointestinal disorders. Neutralizes body odor. Normalizes blood sugar by helping to regulate both hypoglycemia and diabetes.
Garlic	Fights cancer, ulcers, and parasites. Improves the protein levels of blood cells.
Jamaica ginger	Harvested as a small, sprouted plant and then juiced, it helps to regulate the internal thermometer—including slightly elevated temperatures—to combat microbes and mutagens. It also assists in the prevention of motion sickness.
Kale	Rich in calcium and sulfur, it builds bone and acts as a digestive aid and pain reducer.

Mango	Rich in enzymes, it promotes healthy digestion and elimination. Helps build a reserve of vitamins and minerals to create healthy and stable organs.
Mustard	Relieves hemorrhoids, eliminates mucus from the respiratory system, and reduces the term of colds and flu.
Onion	Antimutagenic and anticarcinogenic. Purifies the liver, gall-bladder, spleen, small intestine, and large intestine. Builds immune cells and red blood cells.
Orange	Provides powerful phytonutrients to combat viral and bacterial disease. Assists the neuronal functions of the brain.
Papaya	The high enzyme content encourages gastric, digestive, and pancreatic juices to build blood platelets and reduce external and internal scar tissue.
Quinoa	Harvest and juice these sprouts on the fifth day of sprouting. High protein content and low glycemic properties make this juice a super-fuel that energizes all bodily functions. Increases stamina, strength, and muscle development.
Radish	Increases digestive capability. Reduces fibroid and fibroid cystic growths. Is a powerful antimutagen and anticancer agent.
Red pepper	This juice is a powerhouse of vitamin C and effectively reduces and even prevents viral infections. Helps to prevent blood clots and strokes.
Sweet potato (sprouted leaves)	Builds healthy tissue, compensates for various nutritional deficiencies, and creates elasticity of ligaments.
Tomato	Increases metabolism and reduces excess weight. Reduces fluid in edema. Lycopene and other phytonutrients attack cancers of the prostate, breast, and colon. Combats hepatitis A, B, and C.
Uva-ursi (bearberry)	Eliminates excess mucus and resists microbial infection. It is a diuretic, astringent, mucilage, antiseptic, and disinfectant.
Xanthium (cocklebur)	This antiviral juice helps those with hepatitis A, B, and C, HIV, colds, flu, SARS, and other microbial infections.
Yam (sprouted leaves)	Balances hormones and minimizes the effects of PMS, menopause, mood swings, and low sex drive.
Yucca root (sprouted leaves)	Elevates endurance and energy levels and stimulates the immune function of glycosides to combat all forms of disease.

TABLE 12: *therapeutic vegetable juices*

VEGETABLE JUICE	BENEFITS
Asparagus	Assists renal function, neutralizes kidney stones and bladder stones, and regulates urinary flow.
Artichoke	Enhances the functioning of digestive, immune, and renal systems.
Beet	Consumed in small quantities, it is a blood purifier and blood strengthener. Reduces varicose veins and cleanses arteries and the cardiovascular system.
Brussels sprouts	Contains a protein that helps generate insulin, thereby improving pancreatic function and combating digestive disorders.
Cauliflower	Improves the functioning of skeletal, digestive, and elimination systems.
Celery	Facilitates dermal detoxification and circulation. Reduces uric acid. Improves electrolyte function. Detoxifies the system of the effects of nicotine and caffeine. Promotes dermal flexibility. Provides organic sodium.
Cucumber	Benefits respiratory, renal, joint, and ligament functioning. Increases dermal elasticity.
Daikon radish	Acts as a blood thinner. Maintains electromagnetic functioning of the solar plexus.
Dandelion	Creates red blood cells. Strengthens gums and teeth. Assists healthy bone development (skeletal and dental).
Endive	Improves vision and reduces the potential for and the severity of cataracts. Creates strong ventricular tissue.
Horseradish	Consumed in small amounts, removes excess mucus. Diuretic. Helps to counteract colds and flu.
Iris flower	Builds ligaments, tendons, and cartilage. Strengthens joints and improves membrane development.
Jerusalem artichoke	Stabilizes blood sugar disorders. Generates energy.
Leek	Anticarcinogenic and antimutagenic. Prevents ulcers and inhibits parasites.
Lettuce	A subtle aphrodisiac and mood enhancer. Helps restore hair and skin.
Lily flower	Builds capillaries. Strengthens vision and hearing. Assists the H cell development of the immune system.

Nasturtium	Builds the immune system, fighter cells, and eosinophils. Purifies the lymphatic system and the bloodstream.
Parsley	Minimizes the pain of menstrual cramps. Fights coronary disease, cataracts, conjunctivitis, and glaucoma. Improves vision, cardio-vascular functioning, and blood count.
Pepper (ripe red, yellow, purple)	Reduces bloating, flatulence, colitis, and colic. Rich in vitamin C. Strengthens metabolism, specifically of the heart, and reduces the risk of microbial infection.
Potato (white)	High mineral content, especially potassium, assists renal and cardiovascular function. Effective against arthritic and osteoporotic conditions.
Sauerkraut (raw)	Improves dermal elasticity and appearance. Cleanses and builds the digestive organs. Enhances the probiotics in the gastro-intestinal tract, which in turn strengthen immune cells.
Sorrel	Enhances healthy skeletal and dermal development. Creates greater bone density in the lower extremities.
Spinach	Prevents anemia, convulsions, neuronal disorders, and adrenal dysfunction. Builds red blood cells to cleanse the liver, thereby improving immune function.
String bean (green, purple, yellow)	Regulates blood sugar (in both diabetes and hypoglycemia) by insulin stimulation. Develops proteinase (protein-digesting enzymes).
Tomato	Contains minimal amounts of lycopene. Although it is effective in the reduction of prostate, breast, and colon cancers, and in combating hepatitis A, B, and C, it is less effective than tomato seed sprout juice. Detoxifies the liver and gallbladder.
Turnip greens	Consumed in small quantities, builds bones, facilitates digestion, and prevents colon polyps and hemorrhoids.
Violet flower	Consumed in small quantities, stimulates the spleen and assists in the production of healthy red blood cells, fingernails, and toenails.
Watercress	Consumed in small amounts, increases hemoglobin to prevent anemia and chronic low blood pressure. Strengthens joints, cartilage, tendons, and ligaments. Helps to reduce tumors by improving circulation.
Yellow squash	Packed with bone-building minerals. Acts as a diuretic and relieves constipation.

10 percent fruit juice and 90 percent pure water. For those who are health impaired, it is generally inadvisable to consume any form of fruit juice or the juice of sweet vegetables, such as carrots and beets, because they contain an excess of fructose. The juices of herbs and flowers should be added sparingly, because they have powerful medicinal effects.

When you juice vegetables, fruits, herbs, or flowers, be sure to strain the liquid. At times, given combinations of juices can elevate the desired effect, yielding better results. Even the healthiest person gains significant benefit from the daily consumption of fresh green juices. Two glasses (12 to 16 ounces) of sprouted-vegetable juices taken twice daily are a significant part of the Hippocrates Program. You should consume two ounces of wheat, spelt, kamut, or barley juice—or any combination of these—twice per day. Daily consumption of green juice and grass juice provides your blood and body with the essential nutrients and purification that they require.

People have consumed juices since the beginning of modern civilization. Fresh, raw juices are the best way to acquire needed nutrients in their most digestible form. Energy, strength, cleansing, healing, hydration, and the building and maintenance of the electrolyte system—as well as the renal (kidney) and respiratory systems, the two fluid-based systems of the body—are the main benefits of the consumption of these enzyme-rich liquids.

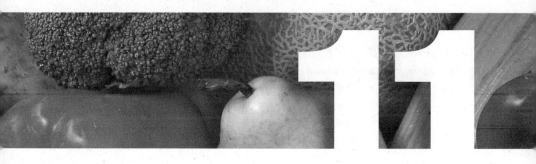

sprouting

health benefits of sprouts

Sprouts are a unique superfood with potent medicinal qualities. They have been a vital dietary resource of the Hippocrates Program since its inception more than half a century ago. Sprouts grown from nuts, seeds, grains, and beans contain ten to thirty times more concentrated nutrients than the most nutritious vegetables. The nutritive value of nuts, seeds, grains, and beans increases more than eight times after germination. Table 13 provides a list of just some of the many delicious, nutritious sprouts you can grow and their health benefits.

TABLE 13: *sprouts and their health benefits*

TYPE OF SPROUT	HEALTH BENEFITS
Apple and apricot	Apple and apricot seeds contain high levels of abscisic acid, a plant hormone and anticancer agent. Scientific evidence indicates that sprouted apple and apricot seeds assist in recovery from all forms of cancer.
Broccoli	Cruciferous vegetables contain a phytonutrient that inhibits the development of cancer. Sprouted broccoli seeds are several dozen times more effective in combating cancer than other vegetables in this family.
Butternut squash	Dried butternut squash seeds germinated in soil produce a succulent green plant (similar to sunflower sprouts) containing nutrients that build the blood and help balance the heart. Cardio-vascular problems may be neutralized by the consumption of butternut squash sprouts and sprouts from other members of the winter squash family in conjunction with a health-supporting lifestyle.
Cabbage	Cabbage sprouts contain anticancer phytochemicals and help battle ulcers and digestive disorders.
Carrot	Carrot tops and sprouted carrot greens are excellent sources of beta-carotene, which benefits vision, healthy pigmentation, and blood purification.
Daikon	The sprouts of the Asian daikon radish yield benefits, unique to the radish family, which include purifying blood, improving circulation, and deterring the development of tumors.
Dill	The consumption of sprouted dill seeds alleviates menstrual problems and helps stabilize blood pressure.
Eucalyptus	Eucalyptus sprouts are very powerful and help combat respiratory and pigment-related disorders.
Fennel	Fennel's ability to build red blood cells and purify the body help to combat clotting problems and breathing disorders.
Fenugreek	Fenugreek sprouts, the heartiest of all sprouts, yield a medicinal gel that helps combat diabetes, digestive disorders, and even body odor.
Garlic	Garlic, a member of the lily family, produces the most antimutagenic, antifungal, and antimicrobial sprout. Its mutagen-fighting capacity is equaled only by that of onions.

Gourds	Conventionally used as seasonal decorations, gourds contain seeds that, when sprouted, produce powerful and positive effects on the body's nervous system and skeletal structure.
Hops	Sprouted hops have a calming effect; they also facilitate the neuron activity of the brain.
Impatiens	The seeds of this edible flower produce sprouts that benefit hair and improve vision.
Jamaica ginger	When this root is planted in organically fertilized soil and watered daily, it sprouts a stalk, which should be consumed before it reaches two inches in height. It helps regulate our internal body temperature to combat microbes and mutagens. It also assists in the prevention of motion sickness.
Jojoba	The sprouted seeds of the fruit of this relatively rare member of the cactus family provide fatty acids for brain tissue development and optimal cardiovascular function; they also help stimulate the immune system's T cells.
Kale	Kale is part of the cruciferous family of vegetables; its significant sulfur and phytonutrient content facilitate cellular function, skeletal repair, and the prevention of cancer.
Kava	Kava seed sprouts help relieve depression without any harmful effect on the liver.
Leeks	Sprouted leeks, which are part of the onion family, benefit the body's respiration, hearing, and glands.
Lima beans	Lima bean sprouts help sustain maximum functioning of the pancreas and kidneys; they also assist in warming the body as necessary.
Mango	The seed within the mango can be dried, placed into soil, and watered twice daily to start the birth of a mango tree. However, to be used as a beneficial sprout, it should be cut and consumed before it reaches two inches in height. The extraordinary enzyme activity in this tropical seed assists weight regulation and cholesterol reduction and inhibits gallbladder malfunction.
Mung beans	Mung bean sprouts (Chinese bean sprouts) are the most easily digestible food; their potent content of zinc, other minerals, and digestible proteins can help prevent prostate problems, glandular dysfunction, and breast cancer, as well as premature balding and graying.

TABLE 13: *sprouts and their health benefits,* continued

TYPE OF SPROUT	HEALTH BENEFITS
Nettle	The seed of the stinging nettle develops by midsummer, and it can be easily found throughout much of the world. Sprouted nettle seeds are among the finest blood purifiers and blood builders in the world of germinated foods.
Nuts	All raw nuts can be sprouted, although you should not sprout or consume peanuts or cashews because they are toxic. For walnuts and pecans, after a lengthy soaking, place the nuts in soil and water them regularly. Eat the shoots before they reach two inches in height. Almonds, hazelnuts, macadamias, pine nuts, and pistachios require overnight soaking. Afterward, place them on an unbleached paper towel, and spray them with pure water at least twice daily. They will be ready to harvest and eat around the third day. All these sprouted nuts, which are rich in protein and essential fatty acids, strengthen the cells, build muscle structure, and sustain the heart.
Onion	Like garlic sprouts, onion sprouts are among the best anticancer foods; they also remove and emulsify pollutants in the organs and circulatory system.
Orange	When dried and sprouted for three days, orange seed sprouts function as an astringent, assisting the removal of bacteria while simultaneously helping white blood cells to cleanse debris from the bloodstream.
Oregano	When sprouted, oregano plant seeds are among the most effective antifungal and antiyeast foods available.
Peas	Pea sprouts, which should be grown on soil for five days, help to build muscle, strengthen teeth, and stimulate H cells.
Poppy seeds	Poppy seeds should be soaked for six hours, then placed on unbleached paper towels and sprayed with pure water at least three times a day. Harvest and eat them on the fourth or fifth day. They are a powerful relaxant and a mood-enhancing food.
Quinoa	The prominent protein content and low glycemic properties of quinoa sprouts make them a super-fuel that energizes all bodily functions, increasing stamina and strength. Quinoa sprouts should be harvested in two days.

Radish	Radish sprouts—which are different from daikon sprouts—facilitate digestion, elimination, and blood cleansing, and they are antimutagenic.
Rye	Rye seed sprouts are beneficial in a several ways: they strengthen the liver and gallbladder, boost energy, and increase sexual potency.
Sesame	Sesame seeds maintain excellent hair, teeth, and bone. These powerful seeds should be soaked for six hours, placed on an unbleached paper towel, sprayed with pure water at least three times per day, and harvested on the fourth day.
Spruce cone	Spruce cone sprouts are created by placing the cone into rich soil, watering it twice a day with warm water, and waiting for the arrival of the baby sprout of the spruce tree. Harvest the sprouts before they are three inches long. Spruce cone sprouts are unique in their ability to strengthen the lungs and enhance brain function.
Sunflower seeds	Sunflower sprouts may be grown on soil or hydroponically in nutritionally enriched pure water for seven days. These sprouts are essential to the Hippocrates Program. They are considered the most balanced of all of the sources of essential amino acids, and they are a perfect source of complete protein. They activate every cell in the immune system, and they build the skeletal, muscular, and neurological systems.
Teff	Teff is a staple of the Ethiopian diet. The sprouts benefit the ventricular, endocrine, and cardiovascular systems.
Tomato	Tomato seed sprouts are remarkable because of their significant phytochemical content. They combat glandular disorders, prostate problems, and breast-related concerns, including cancers.
Uva-ursi (bearberry)	This fascinating plant, a small evergreen shrub, is often called the "upland cranberry." Its seed, dried and then sprouted for three days, is a diuretic, astringent, mucilage, antiseptic, and disinfectant.
Valerian	Valerian sprouts should be consumed in small amounts, as they fuel the nervous system. They can benefit those who suffer from insomnia and should only be consumed before rest or sleep.
Violet flower	Eating violet flower seed sprouts benefits the cardiovascular system and vision, and facilitates neuron activity in the brain.

TABLE 13: *sprouts and their health benefits,* continued

TYPE OF SPROUT	HEALTH BENEFITS
Water chestnut	Water chestnut is a rootlike herb. Planted in soil and watered twice a day, it produces a plant that should be harvested when the attached sprout extending from it is no more than one inch long. It should then be washed and either juiced or sliced into a raw salad. Its ability to strengthen the lungs and kidneys makes it a desirable and delicious part of the diet.
Wild yam	Yam—also known as "China root" and "rheumatism root"—can be planted in soil and watered twice daily to create a sprouted vine. Clip and eat one inch of this sprout. It improves hormone balance and is especially useful for regulating progesterone, estrogen, and DHA. It also eases the functioning of the stomach and bowels, especially when they are inflamed.
Xanthium (cocklebur)	Xanthium is an herb that grows in China, Japan, Korea, Taiwan, and various parts of Europe. Its roots, stems, hairy leaves, and fruits are used in traditional Asian medicine to combat the common cold, headaches, German measles, and other diseases and illnesses. Use the dried seed and sprout it for three days.
Yucca root	Yucca is a starchy root vegetable that should be planted in rich soil and watered twice a day. It will then sprout a green plant that should be harvested before it is three inches tall. The sprouts help elevate endurance and energy levels and stimulate leukocytes (white blood cells), which is an important immune function in the battle against all forms of disease.

a guide to sprouting

After adopting the living food lifestyle, many people initially prefer to purchase their sprouts already grown. The best ones to start with are alfalfa, mung (common "bean sprouts"), chickpea, lentil, mixes of other seeds, sunflower, sweet pea, and fenugreek baby greens.

Eventually, most people who maintain the lifestyle choose to grow their own sprouts to improve the quality and variety of sprouts in their diets or to control the freshness and growing conditions. If you decide to make this jump into self-sufficiency, here are some helpful tips for success. You might also want to consult the following books: *The Sprouting Book* by Ann Wigmore, *Sprouts for the Love of Everybody* by Viktoras Kulvinskas, and *Living Foods for Optimum Health* by Brian Clement.

There are literally thousands of foods that can be sprouted to grow this superior fare. It has been found that playing music during the germinating process can enhance the growth and bounty of food. Research has shown that Mozart's Fifth Symphony is the most stimulating music for the growth of plants. Whether you are present or absent, use this piece or similar works to enhance the development of your plants. Other studies have shown that the same practice, now called the "Mozart effect," enhance the health of humans, including those still in the womb.

Store raw nuts, seeds, grains, beans, and legumes in a sealed container in a cool, dry place (the refrigerator or freezer is best) to lengthen the storage life of these foods prior to sprouting them. Keep in mind that only raw seeds will actually sprout.

TABLE 14: *guidelines for sprouting*

SOAKING

method. Before sprouting nuts, seeds, grains, beans, or legumes, they must be soaked. This helps to eliminate enzyme inhibitors.

Measure the appropriate amount of nuts or seeds and place it into a container. Add at least twice as much water as there are nuts or seeds. Include the recommended amount of MaxiCrop (a brand-name seaweed powder) or an equivalent sea vegetable mixture in the soak water to increase the germination rate.

tips. Starchy seeds, such as grains and legumes, should be soaked in warm water. If nuts or larger seeds must be soaked for more than 12 hours, replace the water with fresh water after the initial 12-hour period. Nuts are ready to be harvested and used after soaking.

SPROUTING

method. Nuts should not be sprouted. To harvest soaked nuts, pour off the soak water, rinse the nuts, and cover them with fresh water before storing them in the refrigerator.

After soaking the seeds for the recommended time, pour off the cloudy water and rinse the seeds as well. During the sprouting process, rinse and drain the growing sprouts every 12 hours. In extreme summer heat, rinse in cool water every 6 hours.

TABLE 14: *guidelines for sprouting,* continued

tips. Place the sprouting container so the soaked seeds stay well drained yet moist, get adequate air, and are kept warm in a dark or semidark location during germination and sprouting.

GREENING

method. Small vegetable seeds are usually used to cultivate chlorophyll after they develop their first two leaves.

tips. Place small seed sprouts in strong indirect sunlight for 1 to 2 days to maximize greening.

HARVESTING

method. Most sprouts and baby greens should be placed into a large bowl of water to wash away the hulls. Grains do not have hulls and do not need to be washed after they have sprouted.

tips. Allow the cleaned sprouts to dry for several hours before putting them in the refrigerator. Sprouted grains do not need to dry and may be placed directly in the refrigerator.

STORAGE

method. Place sprouts into glass or plastic containers lined with paper towels to absorb excess moisture, and store them in the refrigerator. Soaked nuts should be stored in fresh water.

tips. To extend the life of refrigerated sprouts, rinse and drain them every 3 to 4 days. For soaked nuts, change the water every 3 to 4 days. This way sprouts and soaked nuts will last for weeks rather than days.

tips for growing mung bean and adzuki sprouts

For soaking mung and adzuki beans, use very warm soak water (105 to 115 degrees F). If possible, change the soak water several times during the process or keep the soaking seeds in a very hot location.

The secret to long, straight, juicy sprouts is to grow them under pressure in a warm place. One method is to grow them in a colander with a heavy plate on top of them and a weight on top of the plate. This will not squash the sprouts.

growing wheatgrass and baby greens

T
hroughout this book the nutritional benefits of wheatgrass and its juice are extolled based on evidence from scientific studies and the experiences of more than three hundred thousand people who have attended the Hippocrates Lifeforce Program. No sprouting or juicing program can afford to be without wheatgrass. It may be the most healing of all the grasses, with more than one hundred mineral elements from the soil, which help to enhance health. It is certainly one of nature's richest sources of chlorophyll and vitamins A and C, and the juice acts as a purifier of the liver, stomach, pancreas, and circulatory system.

Two other useful and nutritious plants to grow and sprout along with wheatgrass are sunflower baby greens and pea greens. Sunflower greens contain a full spectrum of amino acids (the building blocks of all protein) and a supply of vitamin D, along with abundant sun energy and chlorophyll. Pea greens contain significant amounts of bioactive lecithin and chlorophyll and have been shown to help eliminate plaque deposits, which can build up on the arterial walls.

growing sprouts on trays

SEEDS

buckwheat
(*organically grown*)

sunflower seeds, unhulled
(*organically grown*)

wheat berries
(*organic hard red winter wheat is best*)

SUPPLIES

14" x 18" plastic cafeteria trays

colanders or any container
with drainage holes

MaxiCrop brand seaweed solution

measuring cup

one-gallon containers
(*glass jars work well*)

peat moss

scissors or knife

scoop or hand trowel

spray bottle

topsoil (*organic is best*)

watering can

work gloves

OPTIONAL SUPPLIES

fixtures equipped with full-spectrum lighting

plastic sheeting for under the sprouting rack

rack for growing trays

planting instructions

For each tray, you will need to plant, measure, and soak (but not oversoak) the following quantities of dry seeds in a solution of MaxiCrop and water in one-gallon containers (follow directions on the MaxiCrop bottle). Cover all seeds with at least two inches of the MaxiCrop solution.

2 cups unhulled sunflower seeds

½ cup buckwheat (labeled specifically for sprouting)

¼ cup wheat berries

Soak the seeds for 6 to 8 hours if the ambient temperature is above 70 degrees F. Soak the seeds for 8 to 10 hours if the ambient temperature is below 70 degrees F.

After soaking, drain the seeds into colanders (or other containers with holes in the bottom). Rinse the seeds and let them rest and germinate for 12 to 16 hours. Cover the colanders or containers with clean towels so the seeds will not dry out.

Make a mixture of half topsoil and half peat moss. (Both can be purchased at a nursery or gardening shop.) Fill the trays with this soil mixture. Moisten the soil so it is wet but not soggy. If you over-moisten the soil, leave a narrow trough in the soil near the edge of the trays so excess water can drain into it.

Spread the seeds evenly on the trays. Use about 1¾ cups soaked wheat berries, 2 cups soaked buckwheat, or 2½ cups soaked sunflower seeds per tray.

Mist the seeds with a solution of MaxiCrop and water, and place the trays on a level surface in indirect sunlight or under full-spectrum lighting. A rack with shelves 18 to 24 inches apart is optimal for this purpose.

Optional: Cover the seeds with a thin layer of soil, a plastic bag, or a layer of paper towels for the first 3 days of growing; this helps keep the seeds and soil from drying out. Remove the coverings after 3 days; by this time, the sprouts should be lifting the coverings skyward.

Growing sprouts that are in trays and not covered with plastic should be watered evenly once per day; excess water should be drained 10 minutes after watering. Sunflower greens usually need more water than wheatgrass and buckwheat. Trays covered with plastic need not be watered until the cover is removed.

The trays will be ready to harvest in 7 to 9 days. Harvest your crops with a sharp knife or a pair of scissors. Cut as close to the soil as possible.

sprouting tips

- What if your seeds do not sprout? Either you soaked the seeds too long, or they were already lifeless when you obtained them.

- What if your seeds sprouted but did not grow well? Either the soil was not moist enough or it was too moist, or there was a deficiency in the soil. Use MaxiCrop solution during watering in order to enhance soil nutrition.

- What if there is excess mold? Seeds that do not sprout tend to mold. Either the trays were kept too moist or the seeds were planted too close together and could not breathe. If so, increase air circulation by using a fan or ozone (oxygen-generating) purifier to reduce mold. If the humidity was too high, either a fan or a dehumidifier can be useful. Using plastic bags to cover the seeds and soil for the first three days might cause a problem; if so, try growing the sprouts without them.

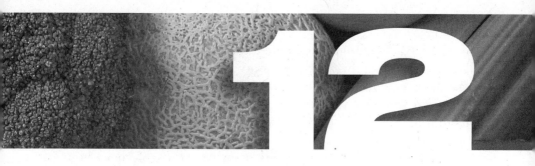

phytochemicals and probiotics

adding phytochemicals to your diet

Phytochemicals, the naturally developing chemicals in all plants, contain compounds that prevent disease and protect our health. More than one thousand families of phytochemicals have been scientifically verified as components of organic, raw living food. Scientists estimate that there are more than one hundred phytochemicals in just one serving of organic vegetables. As early as 1980, the cancer prevention division of the National Cancer Institute began evaluating the effectiveness of phytochemicals in the prevention and treatment of disease. Researchers have known for years that phytochemicals provide self-protection for plants against pests and diseases; now phytochemicals are being studied one by one and are being found useful in protecting humans from disease.

Despite the excitement about the potential of phytonutrients in aiding the prevention of disease, we need to remember that we are still in the infancy of understanding these powerful protectors.

Synthesized compounds that mimic the properties of these natural chemicals do not provide the necessary interaction to fight microbial and mutagenic diseases. Product claims, such as "chemo prevention" and "cancer-preventing nutriceuticals" are used to market man-made "phony phytos" that do not in any way resemble those created by nature.

Most phytonutrient researchers seem barely a step above bean counters, because they are still on a fishing expedition to discover the numbers of these compounds in various plants. They appear to completely disregard the fact that when phytonutrients (phytochemicals) are heated to more than 118 degrees F, their molecular structure is destroyed and they become lifeless microbodies that exist without function. It has even been suggested that more phytochemicals are derived from cooked food than from raw, which is an absurd notion that makes neither common nor scientific sense.

The more than one thousand families of known phytochemicals may be only a fraction of the total that exist in plants. It is astonishing that nature has such a remarkable capacity to provide us with these powerful agents to combat disease and death. Equally remarkable is that some diseases are combated by the phytonutrients derived from plant-based foods that originated millions of years ago, eons before the advent of humans and the diseases we have contracted and created. Think about it—these remedies were actually available before the diseases arrived!

Convincing research continues to show that sprouted beans, grains, nuts, and seeds contain both the greatest cross section and the greatest amounts of these amazing chemicals. Although each of these sources is abundantly capable of growing into a mature plant that produces thousands of still other powerful phytonutrients, you will gain much more from the compact sprouts than from the fully grown plant.

phytochemical food sources

Table 15 lists the most frequently studied of the thousands of phytochemicals that offer benefits to your health. Whenever possible or applicable, sprout the seeds of the following selections to dramatically enhance their phytochemical effects.

TABLE 15: *phytochemicals and their food sources*

PHYTOCHEMICAL	FOOD SOURCES
Carotenoids, phthalides, polyacetylenes	umbelliferous vegetables (carrots, celery, cilantro, parsley, parsnips)
Ellagic acid, phenols, flavonoids (quercetin)	other fruits (apples, berries, cantaloupe, cherries, grapes, pomegranate, watermelon)
Flavonoids (isoflavones), phytic acid, saponins	beans, grains, seeds (barley, brown rice, flaxseeds, mung beans, oats, whole wheat)
Lycopene	solanaceous vegetables (eggplant, peppers, tomatoes)
Monoterpenes (limonene), carotenoids, glucarates	citrus fruits (grapefruit, lemons, oranges)
Silymarin	composite plants (artichokes)

probiotics and homeostatic soil-based organisms

P robiotics and homeostatic soil-based organisms (HSOs) are beneficial strains of microorganisms that generate positive bodily reactions, such as improved bowel function, uninterrupted sleep, enhanced immunity, and noticeably greater amounts of vital energy.

TABLE 16: *beneficial microorganisms*

PROBIOTICS AND HSOS	
Best sources	raw sauerkraut; comprehensive probiotic and/or HSO supplementation.
Symptoms of deficiency	digestive disorders, leaky bowel syndrome, auto-immune disorders, diverticulitis, Crohn's disease, asthma, allergies
Symptoms of toxicity	To date, there is no contraindication for the ingestion of beneficial microorganisms.

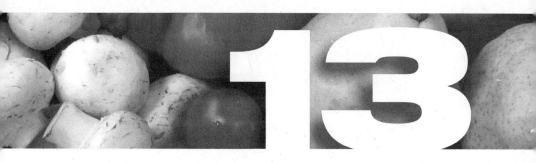

vitamins, protein, fats, and minerals

Charley: "What is it with those vitamins?"

Willy: "They build up your bones. Chemistry."

—FROM ARTHUR MILLER'S
DEATH OF A SALESMAN

During the past several decades, the use of nutritional supplements has become pervasive. Unfortunately, that use has not been accompanied by much concern regarding the sources and applications of nutriceuticals. As a result, approximately 90 percent of man-made nutritional supplements are isolated nutrients generally fabricated by combining petrochemicals with other synthetic chemicals. To sidestep this disturbing trend, we have ever-increasing selections of whole food and whole food derived nutrients that fill the nutritional void created by cooked and processed food.

TABLE 17: *whole food sources of vitamins*

CHOLINE

BEST SOURCES: *broccoli sprouts, cauliflower, grapes, onion sprouts, ripe tomatoes*

MAJOR SYMPTOMS OF DEFICIENCY	MAJOR SYMPTOMS OF TOXICITY
impaired lung functioning	enlargement of the liver and spleen, anemia, increasing physical and mental degeneration

FOLATE folic acid

BEST SOURCES: *beet root greens, broccoli sprouts, lettuce (all kinds), sprouted black-eyed peas, sprouted chickpeas*

MAJOR SYMPTOMS OF DEFICIENCY	MAJOR SYMPTOMS OF TOXICITY
miscarriage, complications of pregnancy, birth defects, neurological malfunction, heart disease	renal toxicity causing kidney enlargement and possible kidney failure

VITAMIN A beta-carotene; retinol

BEST SOURCES: *chia sprouts, cruciferous vegetables, green leafy vegetables, sea vegetables, sunflower green sprouts* (Supplemental vitamin A should be consumed as beta-carotene, which is a precursor of vitamin A.)

MAJOR SYMPTOMS OF DEFICIENCY	MAJOR SYMPTOMS OF TOXICITY
night blindness, dryness of various parts of the eye, blindness	liver damage, irritability, weakness, diminished menstrual bleeding, psychiatric disorders

VITAMIN B₁ thiamin; thiamine

BEST SOURCES: *wheatgrass, raw sauerkraut, sprouted corn, sprouted sweet potatoes, sprouted peas*

MAJOR SYMPTOMS OF DEFICIENCY	MAJOR SYMPTOMS OF TOXICITY
beriberi, headaches, irritability, fatigue, lethargy, neurological diseases	allergic reactions

VITAMIN B₂ riboflavin (formerly cited as vitamin G)

BEST SOURCES: *buckwheat green sprouts, cabbage sprouts, corn sprouts, kamut grass, raw corn, sprouted corn*

MAJOR SYMPTOMS OF DEFICIENCY	MAJOR SYMPTOMS OF TOXICITY
soreness of the mouth and tongue, skin and genital rashes, neuropathy, anemia	possible increase of tumor growth and related complications

VITAMIN B_3 niacin; nicotinamide; nicotinic acid

BEST SOURCES: *dulse, kelp, spelt and kamut grasses, sprouted wheat*

MAJOR SYMPTOMS OF DEFICIENCY	MAJOR SYMPTOMS OF TOXICITY
circulatory and cardiovascular disease	burning, itching, headache, nausea, vomiting, duodenal ulcers, liver failure

VITAMIN B_5 pantothenic acid; calcium pantothenate

BEST SOURCES: *avocado, apricot seeds, organic apples, pecans, sprouted sesame seeds*

MAJOR SYMPTOMS OF DEFICIENCY	MAJOR SYMPTOMS OF TOXICITY
respiratory infection, fatigue, cardiac irregularities, gastrointestinal complications, rashes, staggering, muscle cramps, disorientation	diarrhea, water retention

VITAMIN B_6 pyridoxine; pyridoxal; pyridoxamine

BEST SOURCES: *brussels sprouts, cabbage sprouts, sprouted mango seed, sprouted sweet potatoes, wheatgrass*

MAJOR SYMPTOMS OF DEFICIENCY	MAJOR SYMPTOMS OF TOXICITY
rashes, seizures, carpal tunnel syndrome, anemia	unsteadiness, muscle weakness, systemic weakness

VITAMIN B_{12} (considered a probiotic) cobalamin; cyanocobalamin; hydroxocobalamin

BEST SOURCES: *there are no reliable food sources of vitamin B_{12}; supplementation is necessary*

MAJOR SYMPTOMS OF DEFICIENCY	MAJOR SYMPTOMS OF TOXICITY
pernicious anemia (which sometimes causes unpleasant internal electrical impulses permeating the lips, nose, and extremities), susceptibility to colds and other infections, bruising, impaired blood clotting	allergic reactions; rashes

(continues)

TABLE 17: *whole food sources of vitamins,* continued

VITAMIN C

BEST SOURCES: *black currants, broccoli, cauliflower, kiwifruit, sprouted papaya seed*

MAJOR SYMPTOMS OF DEFICIENCY	MAJOR SYMPTOMS OF TOXICITY
scurvy and its symptoms (primarily spontaneous bleeding), edema and wounds that do not heal, cardiovascular disease, cancer	excessive urination, kidney stones

VITAMIN D

BEST SOURCES: *arame, blue-green algae, clover sprouts, olives, sprouted pinto beans*

MAJOR SYMPTOMS OF DEFICIENCY	MAJOR SYMPTOMS OF TOXICITY
impaired vision, dermal impairment (causing blotches, lack of tautness, and weakness of the skin, hair, and nails)	anemia, weakness, loss of appetite, vomiting, diarrhea, kidney failure, death

VITAMIN E

BEST SOURCES: *avocado, sprouted almonds, sprouted hazelnuts, sprouted pine nuts, sunflower green sprouts*

MAJOR SYMPTOMS OF DEFICIENCY	MAJOR SYMPTOMS OF TOXICITY
anemia, degeneration of the spinal cord and peripheral nerves, weakness	nausea, flatulence, diarrhea, allergic contact dermatitis

VITAMIN H biotin

BEST SOURCES: *hemp seeds, raw sesame tahini, sprouted almonds, sprouted hazelnuts, walnuts*

MAJOR SYMPTOMS OF DEFICIENCY	MAJOR SYMPTOMS OF TOXICITY
disorientation, tremors, loss of memory, speech impairment, unsteady gait, restless legs syndrome	cartilage erosion

VITAMIN K

BEST SOURCES: *alfalfa sprouts, broccoli sprouts, cabbage sprouts, kale, sea kelp*

MAJOR SYMPTOMS OF DEFICIENCY	MAJOR SYMPTOMS OF TOXICITY
blood dilution	blood clotting

At Hippocrates, we conducted a two-year study of the value of nutriceuticals in the processes of self-maintenance and healing. We separated 283 people into two similarly sized groups based on the relative strength or weakness of the cells of their immune systems. These two broadly defined groups consisted of those who were "healthy" and those who were "unhealthy." (Length of illness was not a factor.) The components of each person's physiology that were considered included white blood cells (leukocytes), T cells, H cells, and such differentials as eosinophils, neutrophils, basophils, and lymphocytes. Those who displayed moderate immune strength were placed into the "healthy" group. Those who had abundant immune strength exhibited excellent health, so they too were placed into the same category. In the "unhealthy" group were those who had moderately weak blood test results and those who displayed minimal immune function. We wanted to determine the importance of living, whole food supplements in the recovery and maintenance of the human body. Each participant followed an individually geared nutriceutical program. The study revealed that an average of 26 percent of each "unhealthy" participant's improved immune system functioning resulted from the use of supplements intended for that purpose. This degree of nutritional fulfillment is frequently the difference between life and death, but all too often people wait until they are seriously ill before attempting to improve their lives by stopping self-destructive habits. For the seriously ill, someone who is close to the brink, this successful process might nevertheless be too gradual to generate complete recovery. This is when bioactive, food-based nutrients become essential.

Approximately 7 percent of the immune-building strength of the participants in the "healthy" group was derived from their use of proper supplementation. This seemingly minimal percentage is nevertheless critical to those who use great amounts of energy in their daily activities—people with stressful responsibilities, athletes, those who travel often, and pregnant women. The study also revealed that most of the participants in both groups (at all levels) must consume nutriceutical supplements for approximately two years to regenerate the balance of their immune cells and achieve complete functioning. Adherents of the Hippocrates Lifeforce Program, however, should continue to consume some combination of green and/or blue-green algae on a regular basis.

proteins (amino acids)

Proteins are the building blocks of all life. Many falsehoods exist about protein, primarily that animal products, such as meat, are its best and only complete source. Tables 18 and 19 list the nine essential amino acids and the eleven nonessential amino acids, including the best vegan food sources of each. Please note that many of the foods contain plentiful amounts of most or all of both types of amino acids, and note especially that algae and pollen are uniquely powerful sources

mind-altering and mood-altering proteins

Proteins are also used to enhance psychological states and reduce dependency on conventional psychiatric medicine. Antidepressants, such as Prozac and Zoloft, generate billions of dollars in profits for Eli Lilly and Company and Pfizer Inc., the pharmaceutical companies that manufacture these drugs. However, these medications may induce suicidal thinking and self-harm, and even the United States

TABLE 18: *the nine essential amino acids and their best food sources*

ESSENTIAL AMINO ACIDS	BEST FOOD SOURCES
Histidine	blue-green algae, dulse, lentils, spelt grass
Isoleucine	flower pollen, kelp, mung beans, wakame, wheatgrass
Leucine	freshwater algae, hemp sprouts, hijiki, sesame seeds
Lysine	almonds, green algae, pine nuts, spinach, wheatgrass
Methionine	chickpea sprouts, dulse, flower pollen, kidney bean sprouts
Phenylalanine	sprouted white beans, sunflower green sprouts
Threonine	algae, kamut grass, sesame seeds, sprouted hazelnuts
Tryptophan	kava seeds, sprouted hemp, sprouted squash seeds
Valine	sprouted black-eyed peas, dulse, sunflower green sprouts

TABLE 19: *the eleven nonessential amino acids and their best food sources*

NONESSENTIAL AMINO ACIDS	BEST FOOD SOURCES
Alanine	celery, cranberry seeds, fennel, green algae, sesame seeds
Arginine	black raspberry seeds, celery, kelp , sprouted barley
Asparagine	buckwheat sprouts, sprouted fava beans, turnip greens
Aspartic acid	chia seeds, hijiki, mustard greens, rye sprouts, spinach
Cysteine	blue-green algae, cayenne, kohlrabi, sprouted red beans, sprouted sweet red pepper seeds
Glutamic acid	chlorella, pine nuts, rye grass, sprouted yams
Glutamine	algae, sprouted apple seeds, sprouted cantaloupe seeds
Glycine	hemp seeds, sprouted jicama, sprouted sweet potatoes
Proline	kelp, olives, sprouted lentils, sprouted watermelon seeds
Serine	blue-green algae, flower pollen, sprouted oats, wakame
Tyrosine	dulse, sprouted pear seeds, wheatgrass, winter squash

Food and Drug Administration has been compelled to require the manufacturers to warn consumers of these potential hazards.

Mental exhaustion is often caused by glandular disorders, especially those of the thyroid. L-tyrosine and L-phenylalanine are most often used to combat mental exhaustion and glandular disorders. In cases of physical exhaustion and stress—often caused by adrenal dysfunction—GABA is usually used. In cases of depression, 5-HTP and/or L-tryptophan have proven to be effective in reducing the brain chemistry disorders that cause melancholia and other psychologically depressive conditions.

lipids (fats) and their food sources

L ipids are fatty acids essential to the functioning of both the brain and body. They fuel the immune system and protect us from an entire spectrum of potential disorders.

TABLE 20: *the best food sources of lipids and symptoms of deficiency/toxicity*

LIPIDS	
BEST SOURCES: *Blue-green algae, flaxseed sprouts, hemp seeds, nut sprouts, olives, seed sprouts, sunflower green drink*	
MAJOR SYMPTOMS OF DEFICIENCY	MAJOR SYMPTOMS OF TOXICITY
Attention deficit disorder (ADD), attention deficit hyperactivity disorder (ADHD), digestion and elimination difficulties, irritation of the eyes and skin, neurological dysfunction	Breathing impairment, cardio-vascular problems, rapid weight gain

minerals and trace minerals

M inerals and trace minerals are the circuitry that holds the physical structure of cells together and the energy that fosters hormonal and electrical communication among the cells and other structures of the body. Minerals provide the stability and bonding that are the foundation for all bodily functioning. The absence of minerals and/or trace minerals causes degeneration, susceptibility to disease, and premature aging. Modern scientific technology is constantly revealing new elements, as evidenced by chemistry's constantly changing periodic table of the elements. Thus, new minerals and trace minerals might be discovered at any time. However, the following are and will remain the most significant minerals and trace minerals for the building and maintenance of the human body.

TABLE 21: *minerals and their food sources*

CALCIUM

BEST SOURCES: *dried figs, freshwater algae, green beans, sea algae, sprouted sesame seeds, sprouted sunflower seeds*

MAJOR SYMPTOMS OF DEFICIENCY	MAJOR SYMPTOMS OF TOXICITY
osteoporosis, muscle spasms	constipation, kidney stones, deteriorating renal function

CHROMIUM

BEST SOURCES: *apples, Brazil nuts, mung bean sprouts, rye sprouts, sprouted black-eyed peas, sprouted kidney beans, sprouted watermelon seeds*

MAJOR SYMPTOMS OF DEFICIENCY	MAJOR SYMPTOMS OF TOXICITY
diminished muscle tone, circulatory disorders, heart tissue damage	palpitations, loss of mobility, internal swelling

COPPER (once considered a trace mineral)

BEST SOURCES: *onion sprouts, prunes, shiitake mushrooms, sprouted fenugreek, sunflower green sprouts, turnip greens, wheatgrass*

MAJOR SYMPTOMS OF DEFICIENCY	MAJOR SYMPTOMS OF TOXICITY
anemia, growth impairment, premature graying and/or hair loss	nausea, vomiting, abdominal pain, diarrhea, headache, dizziness, acute poisoning, excessive urination, bone spurs

FLUORIDE (organic)

BEST SOURCES: *garlic, lemons, limes, sprouted radishes, turnip greens*

MAJOR SYMPTOMS OF DEFICIENCY	MAJOR SYMPTOMS OF TOXICITY
erosion of skeletal structure including teeth	anemia, weakness, weight loss, neurological complications, calcification of ligaments

IODINE (also considered a trace mineral)

BEST SOURCES: *arame, dulse, hijiki, kelp, nori*

MAJOR SYMPTOMS OF DEFICIENCY	MAJOR SYMPTOMS OF TOXICITY
goiter, hypothyroidism	thyrotoxicosis

(continues)

TABLE 21: *minerals and their food sources,* continued

IRON

BEST SOURCES: *apricot seeds, arame, dulse, spinach, sprouted barley, sprouted oats, sprouted sesame seeds*

MAJOR SYMPTOMS OF DEFICIENCY	MAJOR SYMPTOMS OF TOXICITY
apathy, attention deficit disorder, irritability, altered immune functioning, anemia, circulatory deficiencies	cardiovascular disease, impaired auto-immune functioning, heart attack, stroke, vulnerability to cancer

MAGNESIUM

BEST SOURCES: *pine nuts, rye sprouts, sprouted pumpkin seeds, sunflower green sprouts, wheatgrass*

MAJOR SYMPTOMS OF DEFICIENCY	MAJOR SYMPTOMS OF TOXICITY
muscle spasms, nausea, vomiting, alterations of personality	nausea, vomiting, diminished blood pressure, diarrhea (Note: magnesium is toxic only to those who have abnormal kidney function.)

MANGANESE

BEST SOURCES: *green coconut water, macadamia nuts, sprouted almonds, sprouted chickpeas, sprouted hazelnuts*

MAJOR SYMPTOMS OF DEFICIENCY	MAJOR SYMPTOMS OF TOXICITY
digestive disorders, lethargy, gastro-intestinal problems	interference with absorption of other minerals and trace minerals, hyper-activity, dilution of blood cells

MOLYBDENUM

BEST SOURCES: *adzuki bean sprouts, green cabbage, spinach, sprouted lentils, sprouted peas*

MAJOR SYMPTOMS OF DEFICIENCY	MAJOR SYMPTOMS OF TOXICITY
increased incidence of esophageal cancer, connective tissue disorder	gout, swollen joints and joint pain, kidney stones, tumors

PHOSPHOROUS

BEST SOURCES: *blue-green algae, chlorella, clover sprouts, dulse, green algae, nori*

MAJOR SYMPTOMS OF DEFICIENCY	MAJOR SYMPTOMS OF TOXICITY
weakness, pain, bone loss, skin irritation, iris impairment	diminished blood calcium levels, cataracts, dryness of the skin causing scaling

POTASSIUM

BEST SOURCES: *green vegetable and sprout juice, parsnip greens, radishes, red peppers, spinach*

MAJOR SYMPTOMS OF DEFICIENCY	MAJOR SYMPTOMS OF TOXICITY
listlessness, drowsiness, fatigue, apprehension, irrational behavior, nausea, vomiting, muscle weakness, spasms, cramps, tachycardia, arrhythmia, diseases and dysfunction of the kidneys, potentially fatal heart failure	kidney failure, acidosis, infections, gastrointestinal hemorrhages, severe muscle trauma, muscle weakness, cardiac irregularities, cardiac failure, death as a result of cardiac arrest, bladder failure, palpitations

SELENIUM (once considered a trace mineral)

BEST SOURCES: *Brazil nuts, grapes, kamut grass, sunflower green sprouts, walnuts*

MAJOR SYMPTOMS OF DEFICIENCY	MAJOR SYMPTOMS OF TOXICITY
mutagenic effects on cells, viruses, weakened immune system, potentially fatal cardiomyopathy	hair loss, nausea, abdominal pain, diarrhea, peripheral neuropathy, fatigue, irritability, hemoglobin coagulation

SILICON

BEST SOURCES: *alfalfa sprouts, beet greens, kamut, oat sprouts, onions, spelt grass, sun tea made from horsetail herb, wheat*

MAJOR SYMPTOMS OF DEFICIENCY	MAJOR SYMPTOMS OF TOXICITY
diminishing elasticity of skin, dry and brittle hair and bones	atherosclerosis

(continues)

TABLE 21: *minerals and their food sources,* continued

SODIUM (organic)	
BEST SOURCES: *celeriac, celery, oat sprouts, sprouted corn, wheatgrass*	
MAJOR SYMPTOMS OF DEFICIENCY	MAJOR SYMPTOMS OF TOXICITY
headaches, muscle weakness	edema, hypertension, congestive heart failure

SULFUR	
BEST SOURCES: *broccoli sprouts, brussels sprouts, cabbage sprouts, garlic sprouts, onion sprouts*	
MAJOR SYMPTOMS OF DEFICIENCY	MAJOR SYMPTOMS OF TOXICITY
increased carbon dioxide in the blood causing lethargy and dizziness	respiratory failure

ZINC	
BEST SOURCES: *broccoli sprouts, brussels sprouts, cabbage sprouts, garlic sprouts, onion sprouts*	
MAJOR SYMPTOMS OF DEFICIENCY	MAJOR SYMPTOMS OF TOXICITY
loss of appetite, anemia, growth retardation, impaired immunity, impaired wound healing, night blindness, photophobia (fear of light), premature graying, hair loss, diminished sense of taste	gastric disturbance, vomiting, impaired immune response

TABLE 22: *trace minerals and their food sources*

MINERAL	MAJOR SYMPTOMS OF DEFICIENCY	MAJOR SYMPTOMS OF TOXICITY
ALUMINUM: *blue-green algae, edible French green clay, string beans*		
	uncontrollable blinking, loss of sensation in the limbs	brain damage, neurological damage, symptoms mimicking Parkinson's disease
ANTIMONY: *celery, chlorella*		
	skin discoloration, impaired vision	disorientation, rashes

MINERAL	MAJOR SYMPTOMS OF DEFICIENCY	MAJOR SYMPTOMS OF TOXICITY
BARIUM: *Ayurvedic supplemental pearl, jicama*		
	constipation, circulatory disorders	cardiovascular problems, reproductive complications
BISMUTH: *dulse, red kidney bean sprouts*		
	eye irritations, impairment of hearing	endocrinal, ovarian, and testicular swelling
BORON: *apple seed sprouts, kelp*		
	skeletal and dental concerns	blood clots, dizziness
BROMINE: *hijiki, ripe pineapples*		
	neurological and/or digestive impairment	unconsciousness
CADMIUM: *dulse, edible French green clay, sea vegetables*		
	impaired vision, loss of memory	paralysis, palpitations
CESIUM: *fermented oat milk*		
	tumorous growths, increased vulnerability to pain	bleeding, stroke
COBALT: *kelp, wheatgrass fertilized with seawater*		
	loss of sensation in the limbs, erupting blood vessels	loss of mobility, including possible paralysis
DEUTERIUM: *arame, ripe tomatoes*		
	endocrinal swelling, palpitations	numbness, pain in the extremities
DYSPROSIUM: *chickpea sprouts, sesame seed sprouts*		
	destruction of leukocytes (white blood cells), which facilitates disease, symptoms of auto-immune malfunction, which may also facilitate disease	liver toxemia, gallbladder toxemia, numbness
ERBIUM: *broccoli sprouts, sauerkraut*		
	gum disease, inflammation of the organs	paralysis, edema

(continues)

TABLE 22: *trace minerals and their food sources,* continued

MINERAL	MAJOR SYMPTOMS OF DEFICIENCY	MAJOR SYMPTOMS OF TOXICITY
EUROPIUM: *figs, pinto bean sprouts*		
	dryness of the skin, impaired capillary functioning	nausea
GADOLINIUM: *barley grass sprouts, dulse, kamut sprouts*		
	intestinal disorders, hormonal imbalance	circulatory disorders, impaired renal functioning
GALLIUM: *fava bean sprouts, lima bean sprouts*		
	digestive disorders, alimentary canal malfunction	gallstones, bladder stones
GERMANIUM: *blue-green algae, European sea vegetables, fenugreek sprouts*		
	autoimmune disease, susceptibility to infection	systemic mineral imbalance
GOLD: *fresh basil, grain grasses grown with seawater*		
	cardiovascular disorder, cartilage deterioration, bone deterioration	paralysis, skeletal erosion
HAFNIUM: *beet greens, broccoli sprouts, kale*		
	respiratory disorders, lung infection including possible pneumonia	skin irritation, glandular impairment
HOLMIUM: *raw macadamia nuts, rye sprouts, turnip seed sprouts*		
	red blood cell reduction, anemia	lightheadedness, unconsciousness
INDIUM: *chlorella, supplemental homeostatic soil organisms (probiotic supplements)*		
	vision impairment, hearing impairment	joint pain, dizziness
IRIDIUM: *alfalfa, apricot seeds*		
	diminished hemoglobin count causing lethargy, circulatory disorders	weakness, fever
LANTHANUM: *collard greens, fava bean sprouts*		
	muscular weakness, joint pain	paralysis, psychological degeneration

MINERAL	MAJOR SYMPTOMS OF DEFICIENCY	MAJOR SYMPTOMS OF TOXICITY
LITHIUM: *adzuki sprouts, fresh herbal hops*		
	hallucinations, insecurity	disorientation, liver failure
LUTETIUM: *arugula, celery, raw macadamia nuts*		
	hair, nail, and skin impairment	excess production of tears, neurological distress
NICKEL: *kale, mustard seed sprouts*		
	respiratory impairment, blurred vision	paralysis, numbness
NIOBIUM: *black mission figs, hazelnut sprouts*		
	lymphatic dysfunction, reproductive dysfunction	dizziness, susceptibility to colds and flu
OSMIUM: *nori, sprouted sweet potatoes*		
	impairment of tissue density	internal bleeding
PALLADIUM: *coastal-grown vegetables, green coconuts*		
	paralysis, mental impairment, psychological dysfunction	respiratory impairment
PLATINUM: *arame, kelp*		
	weakening of heart tissue, ventricular collapse	paralysis, neurological dysfunction
PRASEODYMIUM: *broccoli sprouts, rutabagas*		
	arthritis, tooth decay	nausea
RHENIUM: *black currants, chickpea sprouts*		
	bladder malfunction, renal failure	excess perspiration, excess urination
RUBIDIUM: *fresh thyme, sprouted green juice*		
	vision impairment, rashes	palpitations
RUTHENIUM: *garlic, garlic sprouts, mustard seed sprouts*		
	circulatory impairment possibly causing dysfunction of limbs and/or organs, indigestion	stroke, weakened muscular structure

(continues)

TABLE 22: *trace minerals and their food sources,* continued

MINERAL	MAJOR SYMPTOMS OF DEFICIENCY	MAJOR SYMPTOMS OF TOXICITY
SAMARIUM: *dandelion, hijiki, nettle*		
	bowel disorders, gallstones	gas and bloating, lethargy
SILVER: *lamb's-quarters herb, nori*		
	arrhythmia, microbial infections	paralysis, brain impairment
STRONTIUM: *black-eyed pea sprouts, green peas*		
	limited circulation in the extremities	muscle weakness, exhaustion
TANTALUM: *green pea sprouts, lima bean sprouts, mangoes*		
	skin irritation, blood clots	weakness, excessive stress
TIN: *chlorella, Great Northern bean sprouts*		
	renal weakness, respiratory dysfunction	exhaustion, weakened extremities
TUNGSTEN: *barley, Brazil nut sprouts, mung bean sprouts*		
	weakened spleen, arrhythmia	anemia
VANADIUM: *clover sprouts, nasturtium flowers, walnuts*		
	impaired circulation, vision impairment	fever, hot flashes
ZIRCONIUM: *red bean sprouts, sprouted mango seeds, sprouted yams*		
	respiratory inflammation, irritation of the eyes	dizziness, nausea

14

medicinal herbs

Medicinal herbs are used by most of the world's population as their main source of medicine. People in Western cultures use mostly modern pharmaceuticals. However, approximately one-fourth of all pharmaceutical medicines consist exclusively of herbs, and, with the exception of nuclear medicine, all pharmaceuticals have plant-based origins.

Throughout human history, various schools of herbology have developed around the world. Most respected among them is the internationally esteemed Asian tradition, which spans several thousand years. The practitioners of this well-documented science have demonstrated that every ailment has one or more natural antidotes. The origins of herbal medicine can be traced to the African continent; unfortunately, both that history and Native American herbology are almost completely lost because of shameful abuse of those populations and brutal disregard for their traditions and artifacts. Health and healing have specific histories based on geography and culture. The residents of each region and each individual group cultivated their own medicinal systems to combat disease.

The variety of herbs available internationally is extensive. For example, throughout Europe, those healing plants found in the north—for example, Lapland—are uniquely different from those harvested in southern Spain. And there are hundreds of varieties of medicinal herbs in Australia that are unique to that continent. In South America and the islands of the South Pacific, plentiful herbs are used for nutrition and health.

Despite these well-documented traditions, in Western medicine the use of herbs was relegated to the status of "alternative treatment" and lost its historically validated prominence as our primary remedy. In addition, many people segregate pharmaceuticals from herbal medicines, falsely believing that they can use herbs without concern or restriction. The fact is that herbs are medicine and therefore must be given the same consideration and utilized with the same discipline as pharmaceuticals. (We do acknowledge the distressing fact that pharmaceuticals are very frequently used inappropriately, excessively, and criminally.)

It is potentially extremely dangerous to combine herbal medicines, combine herbal medicines and pharmaceuticals, or combine various pharmaceuticals. Overuse, misuse, and abuse of pharmaceuticals are not only serious problems but the foremost basis of criticism of the frequent irresponsible prescription of these substances. Inappropriate use of prescription medications is often the cause of both symptoms and disorders. Pharmaceutical medicine does, of course, serve a valuable purpose, so it is neither to be disregarded nor dismissed. It must be properly used, but only after all herbal medicinal options—the most natural means of healing—have been considered, and only in conjunction with the counsel of an experienced, competent practitioner.

Those who manufacture herbs often mislead consumers unintentionally by neglecting to mention a critical fact: habitual use of some herbal substances can be detrimental to their health. We should rarely consume any herb for long periods. There are a few exceptions, for example natural hormones for women, ginkgo biloba for cranial and ventricular problems, and cranberry extracts for kidney infections, bladder problems, and long-term complications. Please note that some seasonings and herbs, such as mint, oregano, chamomile, and others, are not dangerous, even if they are used regularly as condiments throughout a lifetime. Exceptions include various salts and black pepper.

For those who use medicinal herbs, the Hippocrates Institute has established a safe pattern of consumption: Take medicinal herbs for three days, and then do not take them for the next three days; in addition, do not take them at all every eighth week. This sequence provides you with better results than habitual use, because constant supplemental support of the body's natural chemistry increases the need for additional supplementation, thereby reducing the effectiveness of any given herb.

Commonly used herbs, such as echinacea, are best utilized at the time you are exposed to an infection. Echinacea is of little or no value once an infection has taken hold. After you have been infected, an herb such as osha or the temporary use of silver nitrate (colloidal silver) is preferable. Aloe vera can be used daily, because it is in the rare category of medicinal food herbs, meaning that it is both a food and a medicine. Conversely, cayenne, which is also a medicinal food herb, should not be consumed in large amounts over a long period because it is extremely potent.

Seasons and altitudes are as important to herbs as they are to the availability of certain plants. For example, nettle is found throughout the world, but it develops only during spring. Its blood-purifying properties are welcome after a long, dark winter. Certain cool-weather plants, such as dandelion flower, grow only at the cooler, higher altitudes during extreme summer; therefore, residents at those altitudes can harvest them for their blood-building benefits. And many herbs can be consistently found at both higher and lower altitudes.

Consuming fresh raw herbs is always preferable, but seasonal restrictions often leave us with the sole choice of using them dried. When dried herbs are used, it is best to make a sun tea from them. Use at least one teaspoon of dried herbs for each cup of pure water; more herbs may be used for a stronger tea. Place the container on a windowsill for twenty-four hours, making sure that the window remains closed. After this one-day process, you can warm the herbal tea, taking care that you do not heat it above 115 degrees F. There are exceptions to these instructions for consuming herbs: Dried or gelatin-free encapsulated powders and herbal pills that have not been heated during manufacture are also possibilities. The addition of small amounts of herbs to your fresh juices will enhance the already powerful effects of these beneficial and nutritious liquids. For example, the juiced combination of fresh ginger and green vegetables assists the digestion of their nutrients, regulates the thermostat of the human body, and calms the stomach and intestines.

When you buy processed herbs, try to find those that are both liquid and in glycerin. These extracts are potentially more potent and much more digestible than other forms; they are also preserved by the glycerin, which protects their medicinal fluids from oxidization, which results in loss of potency.

TABLE 23: *selected list of medicinal herbs*

MEDICINAL HERBS	BEST SOURCES	ATTRIBUTED MEDICINAL RELIEF
Angelica	fresh root, leaf	respiratory, bronchial, antiviral
Basil	fresh leaf	mild sedative, antiseptic, relieves nausea
Catnip	fresh leaf	colds, catarrh, bronchitis
Dandelion	fresh root, leaf	liver maintenance, diuretic, laxative, juice combats warts
Elder	root, stem, leaf	coughs, catarrh, rheumatism, sciatica, combats cysts
Feverfew	complete plant	headaches, migraines, natural insect repellent
Geranium	plant or flower	cardiovascular benefits
Horseradish	root	benefits lungs and circulation, blood cleanser
Iris	fresh flower	ligaments, tendons, joints, cartilage, membrane development
Juniper	berry, leaf	digestion, renal function, blood cleanser
Kohlrabi	root, stem, leaf	antimutagenic, ulcers, digestion
Lavender	flower, leaf	antiseptic, equilibrium, rheumatism, relaxant
Marigold	stem, flower	heals wounds, conjunctivitis, bee and wasp stings
Nettle	root, stem, leaf	arthritis, internal bleeding, skin conditions, detoxification
Orris	root, leaf	throat infection, bladder problems
Pennyroyal	stem, leaf, flower	flatulence, nausea, headaches
Quinoa	root, plant	builds red blood cells, strengthens neurological system
Rue	seed, root, leaf, stem, flower	epilepsy, eczema, psoriasis, ointment for eyes and throat
Sorrel	stem, leaf	diuretic, kidney tonic
Tarragon	stem, leaf	toothache, antimutagenic

MEDICINAL HERBS	BEST SOURCES	ATTRIBUTED MEDICINAL RELIEF
Uva-ursi (bearberry)	root, leaf	backache, bladder congestion, renal congestion, prostate, gonorrhea, syphilis
Valerian	root, stem, leaf	sedative, tranquilizer, insomnia, nerve disorders
Wallflower	stem, leaf	cardiovascular functioning, arterial elasticity
Xanthium (cocklebur)	seed	hepatitis, colds, flu, SARS, other microbial infections
Yarrow	stem, leaf, flower	diarrhea, dysentery, astringent
Zingiber	root	combats microbes and mutagens, controls elevated temperature, prevents motion sickness

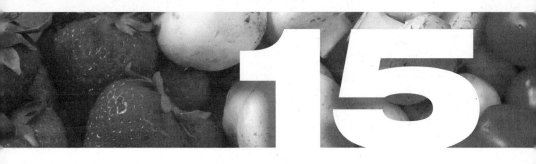

equipment and resources

equipment

Some kitchen items are essential if you wish to incorporate the living food program into your daily routine. For instance, a dehydrator will allow you to produce your own snacks, dried fruit, crackers, and other foods that will help you maintain a high-quality diet.

Sprouting supplies can be relatively inexpensive, while juicers and dehydrators cost quite a bit more. Below is a list of essential items and some that are optional but highly recommended. All of the supplies and equipment can be obtained from the Hippocrates Health Institute online at www.hippocratesinstitute.com or by calling 561-471-8876, ext. 124.

- automatic sprouter (optional)
- blender
- body slant cushion (optional)
- dry skin brush
- electric seed mill (optional)
- enema bag with catheter, wheatgrass syringe, bulb for wheatgrass syringe

- food dehydrator (Excalibur brand is recommended)
- food processor (optional)
- home distiller
- home water filter
- planting supplies (trays, seeds)
- portable water filter for travel (optional)
- sprouting supplies (jars, bags, seeds, mesh)
- vegetable juicer
- wheatgrass juicer, preferably electric

resources

Numerous Web sites provide information about organic, vegan, and raw food, including suppliers and other resources such as restaurants, markets, individual growers, and food co-ops. The following is not a comprehensive list. For the most up-to-date listings, use your favorite search engine and type in "raw food restaurants," "living food resources," "vegan worldwide restaurants," or "wheatgrass delivery."

Door to Door Organics

www.doortodoororganics.com

Door to Door Organics is based on the east coast of the United States and has been delivering farm fresh organic produce to homes and offices since 1996. They deliver to nine states and the District of Columbia. Wheatgrass, both live and cut, is one of their specialties.

GreenPeople

www.greenpeople.org

GreenPeople bills itself as the world's largest directory of ecofriendly and holistic health products. From organic vegan food and organic clothes to chemical-free cleaning products, this site is the one-stop place to shop.

LocalHarvest

www.localharvest.org

LocalHarvest features a search engine you can use to find local organic food farms, markets, grocers, and restaurants within your area. Listings even come in categories such as specific types of vegetables or organic personal care products. An events calendar keeps track of occasions when like-minded people come together to celebrate the organic way of life.

Natural Food Network

www.naturalfoodnet.com

The directory of certified-organic food on this site will help you find organic food suppliers throughout North America. News stories and research data on natural food are also regular features of this Web site.

Pines International

www.wheatgrass.com

Pines International grows and distributes fresh wheatgrass and related products.

Raw Food Life

www.rawfoodlife.com

You will find good information about the raw food diet in general on this site, as well as research about the dangers of cooked food.

SoyStache

www.soystache.com

Dozens of raw food restaurants throughout North America are listed and linked on this Web site.

SuperMarketCoop

www.supermarketcoop.com

SuperMarketCoop hosts rural, community-based agricultural cooperatives that provide more wholesome alternatives to what is typically found in chain supermarkets. A co-op directory enables you to search for growers serving the United States and Mexico.

VegDining.com

www.vegdining.com

VegDining.com is an online guide to vegetarian restaurants. The site will enable you to locate suitable dining establishments around the world.

Vegetarian Resource Group

www.vrg.org

The Vegetarian Resource Group's Web site has everything from recipes to listings of natural food restaurants and grocery outlets.

other useful web sites

www.fredericpatenaude.com

www.howtogoraw.com

www.livingnutrition.com

www.rawfoodnews.com

references

introduction

Centers for Disease Control and Prevention. "Prevalence of Autism Spectrum Disorders." *Morbidity and Mortality Weekly Report* 56 (February 9, 2007). http://www.cdc.gov/mmwr/pdf/ss/ss5601.pdf.

National Center for Health Statistics. "Deaths/Mortality." http://www.cdc.gov/nchs/fastats/deaths.htm.

National Coalition on Health Care. "Facts on the Cost of Health Care." http://www.nchc.org/facts/cost.shtml.

National Institute of Diabetes and Digestive and Kidney Diseases. "Statistics: Diabetes." http://diabetes.niddk.nih.gov/populations/index.htm.

Ries, L. A. G., M. P. Eisner, C. L. Kosary, B. F. Hankey, B. A. Miller, L. Clegg, A. Mariotto, E. J. Feuer, and B. K. Edwards, eds. "SEER Cancer Statistics Review, 1975_2002." National Cancer Institute. Bethesda, MD. http://seer.cancer.gov/csr/1975–2002. Based on November 2004 SEER data submission, posted to the SEER Web site 2005.

Schieve, L. A., C. Rice, C. Boyle, S. N. Visser, and S. J. Blumberg. "Mental Health in the United States: Parental Report of Diagnosed Autism in Children Aged 4–17 Years—United States, 2003–2004." *Morbidity and Mortality Weekly Report* 55, no. 17 (2006): 481–486. http://www.cdc.gov/mmwr/preview/mmwrhtml/mm5517a3.htm.

"Vallombrosa Consensus Statement on Environmental Contaminants and Human Fertility Compromise." October 2005. http://obgyn-nw.ucsf.edu/docs/Vallombrosa_Consensus_Statement.pdf.

World Health Organization. "Basic Health Information on Nutrition." March 13, 2006. http://www.wpro.who.int/information_sources/databases/regional_statistics/rstat_nutrition.htm.

World Health Organization. "Global Burden of Cancer in the Year 2000." August 15, 2006. http://www.who.int/healthinfo/statistics/bod_malignantneoplasmscancers.pdf.

chapter 1

Associated Press. "Obesity: Small Steps Help." *CBS News*, May 30, 2004. http://www.cbsnews.com/stories/2004/05/30/health/main620334.shtml.

Cancer Research UK. "Diet and Cancer: The Story So Far." May 18, 2004. http://info.cancerresearchuk.org/news/pressreleases/2004/may/38889.

———. "Vanity Beats Cancer as Motivation for Weight Loss." August 9, 2006. http://info.cancerresearchuk.org/news/pressreleases/2006/august/vanity beatscancer.

Ennis, Darren. "Half of Europe Fat but Sees No Health Threat." *Reuters*, February 28, 2006.

Hales, Dianne. "We're Changing the Way We Eat." *Parade*, November 12, 2006.

Halton, Thomas L., et. al. "Low-Carbohydrate-Diet Score and the Risk of Coronary Heart Disease in Women." *The New England Journal of Medicine* 355, no. 19 (November 9, 2006): 1991–2002.

Moss, Lyndsay. "Children Doomed to Obesity by 'Toxic, Addictive' Fast-Food." *Scotsman*, August 12, 2006.

Petersen, M. et. al., "Randomized, Multi-center trial of Two Hypo-energetics Diets in Obese Subjects: High versus Low Fat Content." *International Journal of Obesity*. 30 (March 2006): 552–560.

Saul, Stephanie. "Two Approaches to the Nation's Obesity Epidemic Coming Up for Review." *New York Times*, January 17, 2006.

Sullivan, Rohan. "Health Experts: Obesity Pandemic Looms." *Associated Press*, September 3, 2006.

chapter 2

Associated Press. "Women Told They Have Math Abilities Equal to Men Get More Right Answers." October 19, 2006.

BBC News. "Positive Thinking a Pain Reliever." September 5, 2005.

Jerusalem Post. "Study: Most Doctors Use Placebos." September 19, 2004.

Motluk, Alison. "Placebo Produces Surprise Biological Effect." *New Scientist*, August 9, 2001. http://www.newscientist.com/article.ns?id=dn1137.

Reid, Brian. "The Nocebo Effect: Placebo's Evil Twin." *Washington Post*, April 30, 2002.

Young, Emma. "Brain Scans Reveal Placebo Effect in Depressed Patients." *New Scientist*, January 2, 2002. http://www.newscientist.com/article.ns?id=dn1732.

chapter 3

BBC News. "Food Chemicals May Harm Humans." September 9, 2006.

Clapp, Richard, Genevieve Howe, and Molly Jacobs Lefevre. "Environmental and Occupational Causes of Cancer." Prepared by Boston University School of Public Health and the Environmental Health Initiative, University of Massachusetts Lowell. Lowell, MA: Lowell Center for Sustainable Production, September 2005.

Duncan, David Ewing. "The Pollution Within." *National Geographic*, October 2006.

Environment News Service. "Chemicals Found in Common European Foods." September 21, 2006. http://www.ens-newswire.com/ens/sep2006/ 2006-09-21-02.asp.

Environmental Working Group. "Across Generations: The Chemical Pollution Mothers and Daughters Share and Inherit." May 10, 2006. http://www.ewg.org/reports/generations.

Greenpeace and World Wildlife Fund. "A Present for Life: Hazardous Chemicals in Umbilical Cord Blood." September 2005.

Laurance, Jeremy. "Chemical Pollution Harms Children's Brains." *Independent*, November 9, 2006.

Lawrence, Felicity. "Omega-3, Junk Food and the Link between Violence and What We Eat." *Guardian*, October 17, 2006.

Montague, Peter. "Why We Can't Prevent Cancer." *Rachel's Democracy and Health News*, October 27, 2005.

Our Stolen Future Web site. "Emerging Science on the Impacts of Endocrine Disruption on Reproduction and Fertility." http://www.ourstolenfuture.org/newscience/reproduction/repro.htm

Paulson, Tom. "Startling Study on Toxins' Harm." *Seattle Post-Intelligencer*, June 3, 2005.

chapter 4

Bowers, W. F. "Chlorophyll in Wound Healing and Suppurative Disease." *American Journal of Surgery* 73 (1947): 37–50.

Gaisbauer, M., and A. Langosch. "Raw Food and Immunity." *Fortschritte der Medizin* 108, no. 17 (June 10, 1990): 338–340.

"Leukocytosis and Cooked Versus Raw Foods." *Proceedings of the First International Congress of Macrobiology*. Paris, 1930.

Manoukian, R., M. Citton, P. Huerta, B. Rhode, C. Drapeau, and G. S. Jensen. "Effects of the Blue-Green Algae *Aphanizomenon flos-aquae* (L.) Ralphs on Human Natural Killer Cells." In *Phytoceuticals: Examining the Health Benefits and Pharmaceutical Properties of Natural Antioxidants and Phytochemicals*, edited by L. Savage. IBC Library Series, vol. 1911, chap. 3.1, pp. 233–241, 1998.

Messaoudi, I., J. Warner, M. Fischer, B. Park, B. Hill, J. Mattison, M. A. Lane, et al. "Delay of T Cell Senescence by Caloric Restriction in Aged Long-Lived Non-human Primates." *Proceedings of the National Academy of Sciences* 103, no. 51 (2006): 19448–19453.

MSNBC. "Does Your Heart Sense Your Emotional State? Stressful Feelings May Increase Your Risk of Developing Heart Disease." January 26, 2006. http://www.msnbc.msn.com/id/11023208.

"Non-meat Eaters, Longevity and Chronic Health Disorders." *Journal of the American Medical Association* 176 (1961): 803.

Offenkrantz, W. G. "Water-Soluble Chlorophyll in the Treatment of Peptic Ulcers of Long Duration." *Review of Gastroenterology* 17, no. 5 (May 1950): 359–367.

Rafsky, K. "Treatment of Intestinal Disease with Solutions of Water-Soluble Chlorophyll." *Review of Gastroenterology* 15 (1948): 549.

Silveira, E. M., M. F. Rodrigues, M. S. Krause, D. R. Vianna, B. S. Almeida, J. S. Rossato, L. P. Oliveira, R. Curi, and P. I. H. de Bittencourt. "Acute Exercise

Stimulates Macrophage Function." *Cell Biochemistry and Function* 25, no. 1 (2007): 63–73.

Tannenbaum, A. "Nutrition and Cancer." In *The Physiopathology of Cancer*, 2nd ed., edited by F. Homburger, 517–562. New York: Hoeber-Harper, 1959.

chapter 5

Angier, Natalie. "Researchers Find a Concentrated Anticancer Substance in Broccoli Sprouts." *New York Times*, September 16, 1997.

Annand, J. C. "Thrombosis: Further Evidence Against Heated Animal Protein." *Journal of the College of General Practitioners* 20 (1964): 386–401.

———. "Vegetable Consumption and Heart Disorders." *Journal of the College of General Practitioners* 2 (1959): 365.

Associated Press. "Diabetes Drug's Benefits Come at a Price." December 4, 2006.

Banerjee, D. K., and J. B. Chatterjea. "Vitamin B_{12} Content of Some Articles of Indian Diets and Effect of Cooking on It." *British Journal of Nutrition* 17 (1963): 385–389.

Barnard, N. D., J. Cohen, D. J. Jenkins, G. Turner-McGrievy, L. Gloede, B. Jaster, K. Seidl, A. A. Green, and S. Talpers. "A Low-Fat Vegan Diet Improves Glycemic Control." *Diabetes Care* 29 (2006): 1777–1783.

BBC News. "High-Veg Diet Wards Off Cancer." December 24, 2005.

Collins, Karen. "Magical Food Combos That Fight Cancer." *Bottom Line/Personal*, February 1, 2007.

Fahey, J. W., X. Haristoy, P. M. Dolan, T. W. Kensler, I. Scholtus, K. K. Stephenson, P. Talalay, and A. Lozniewski. "Sulforaphane Inhibits Extracellular, Intracellular, and Antibiotic-Resistant Strains of *Helicobacter pylori* and Prevents Benzo[a]pyrene-Induced Stomach Tumors." *Proceedings of the National Academy of Sciences* 99, no. 11 (2002): 7610–7615.

Fontana, L., J. L. Shew, J. O. Holloszy, and D. T. Villareal. "Low Bone Mass in Subjects on a Long-Term Raw Vegetarian Diet." *Archives of Internal Medicine* 165 (March 28, 2005): 684–689.

Hanninen, O., K. Kaartinen, A. L. Rauma, M. Nenonen, R. Torronen, A. S. Hakkinen, H. Adlercreutz, and J. Laakso. "Antioxidants in Vegan Diet and Rheumatic Disorders." *Toxicology* 155, nos. 1–3 (November 30, 2000): 45–53.

Healy, Z. R., N. H. Lee, X. Gao, M. B. Goldring, P. Talalay, T. W. Kensler, and K. Konstantopoulos. "Divergent Responses of Chondrocytes and Endothelial Cells to Shear Stress: Cross-Talk among COX-2, the Phase 2 Response, and Apoptosis." *Proceedings of the National Academy of Sciences* 102 (September 27, 2005): 14010–14015.

Institute of Food Research. "Can Our Diet Protect Us Against Cancer?" http://www.ifr.ac.uk/Public/FoodInfoSheets/diet_and_cancer.html.

Kage, Ben. "Mineral Depletion of Soils Results in Higher Acrylamide Content of Foods." NewsTarget.com, November 13, 2006. http://www.newstarget.com/021053.html.

Laurance, Jeremy. "Miracle Cures Shown to Work." *Independent*, January 23, 2006.

Ling, W. H., and O. Hanninen. "Shifting from a Conventional Diet to an Uncooked Vegan Diet Reversibly Alters Fecal Hydrolytic Activities in Humans." *Journal of Nutrition* 122, no. 4 (April 1992): 924–930.

Linus Pauling Institute. "Fighting Cancer with Phytochemicals: An Interview with David E. Williams, Ph.D." *LPI Research Newsletter*, Fall 2006. http://lpi.oregon-state.edu/fw06/phytochemicals1.html.

————. "Indole-3-Carbinol: Effects of Cooking." Oregon State University. July 21, 2005. http://lpi.oregonstate.edu/infocenter/phytochemicals/ i3c/index.html.

London, S. J., J.-M. Yuan, F.-L. Chung, Y.-T. Gao, G. A. Coetzee, R. K. Ross, and M. C. Yu. "Isothiocyanates, Glutathione S-transferase M1 and T1 Polymorphisms, and Lung-Cancer Risk: A Prospective Study of Men in Shanghai, China." *Lancet* 356 (August 26, 2000): 724–729.

McDonald, L., and M. Edgill. "Dietary Restriction and Coagulability of the Blood in Ischæmic Heart-Disease." *Lancet* 271, no. 7028 (1958): 996–998.

Nicholson, A. S., M. Sklar, N. D. Barnard, S. Gore, R. Sullivan, and S. Browning. "Toward Improved Management of NIDDM: A Randomized, Controlled Pilot Intervention Using a Lowfat Vegetarian Diet." *Preventive Medicine* 29, no. 2 (1999): 87–91.

Peltonen, R., M. Nenonen, T. Helve, O. Hanninen, P. Toivanen, and E. Eerola. "Faecal Microbial Flora and Disease Activity in Rheumatoid Arthritis During a Vegan Diet." *British Journal of Rheumatology* 36, no. 1 (1997): 64–68.

Reuters. "Broccoli May Help Bladder Cancer." August 3, 2005.

Smith, T. K., E. K. Lund, M. L. Parker, R. G. Clarke, and I. T. Johnson. "Allyl-isothiocyanate Causes Mitotic Block, Loss of Cell Adhesion and Disrupted Cytoskeletal Structure in HT29 Cells." *Carcinogenesis* 25, no. 8 (2004): 1409–1415.

Stein, Rob. "Breast Cancer Study Suggests Red Meat Link." *Washington Post*, November 14, 2006.

Trock, B., E. Lanza, and P. Greenwald. "Dietary Fiber, Vegetables, and Colon Cancer: Critical Review and Meta-analyses of the Epidemiologic Evidence." *Journal of the National Cancer Institute* 82 (1990): 650–661.

Walker, G. R., E. H. Morse, and V. A. Overley. "The Effect of Animal Protein and Vegetable Protein Diets Having the Same Fat Content on the Serum Lipid Levels of Young Women." *Journal of Nutrition* 72 (November 1960): 317–321.

Yamamoto, I., T. Nagumo, K. Yagi, H. Tominaga, and M. Aoki. "Antitumor Effect of Seaweeds." *Japanese Journal of Experimental Medicine* 44, no. 6 (1974): 543–546.

Yochum, L., L. H. Kushi, K. Meyer, and A. R. Folsom. "Dietary Flavonoid Intake and Risk of Cardiovascular Disease in Postmenopausal Women." *American Journal of Epidemiology* 149 (May 15, 1999): 943–949.

chapter 6

American Society of Integrative Medical Practice. "Report Card on America's Health, 2006–2026." June 10, 2006. http://www.asimp.org.

Associated Press. "Research Shows Low-Calorie Diet May Lead to Longer Life." April 5, 2006.

BBC News. "Juices May Cut Alzheimer's Risk." August 31, 2006.

Geiger, Debbe. "Healthy Hints from Okinawa for Good Living Past 100." *Newsday,* July 23, 2001.

Jenkins, D., C. Kendall, D. Faulkner, T. Nguyen, T. Kemp, A. Marchie, J. Wong, et al. "Assessment of the Longer-Term Effects of a Dietary Portfolio of Cholesterol-Lowering Foods in Hypercholesterolemia." *American Journal of Clinical Nutrition* 83 (March 2006): 582–591.

Kurkella, R. "Cooked Fats and Premature Death in Animals." *Zusammen faasiender Vortrag mit Literaturangaben* no. 3 (1968): 57–65.

Maher, P., T. Akaishi, and K. Abe. "Flavonoid Fisetin Promotes ERK-Dependent Long-Term Potentiation and Enhances Memory." *Proceedings of the National Academy of Sciences* 103, no. 44 (2006): 16568–16573.

Olaharski, A. J., J. Rine, B. L. Marshall, J. Babiarz, L. Zhang, E. Verdin, and M. T. Smith. "The Flavoring Agent Dihydrocoumarin Reverses Epigenetic Silencing and Inhibits Sirtuin Deacetylases." *Public Library of Science (PLoS) Genetics* 1, no. 6 (December 2005): e77.

Qin, W., M. Chachich, M. Lane, G. Roth, M. Bryant, R. de Cabo, M. A. Ottinger, et al. "Calorie Restriction Attenuates Alzheimer's Disease Type Brain Amyloidosis in Squirrel Monkeys (*Saimiri sciureus*)." *Journal of Alzheimer's Disease* 10, no. 4 (December 2006): 417–422.

Reinberg, Steven. "The Smarter They Are, the More Likely They'll Shun Meat as Adults." *HealthDay News,* December 15, 2006.

Schlenker, E. D., J. S. Feurig, L. H. Stone, M. A. Ohlson, and O. Mickelsen. "Nutrition and Health of Older People." *American Journal of Clinical Nutrition* 26, no. 10 (1973): 1111–1119.

Spector, I. M. "Animal Longevity and Protein Turnover Rate." *Nature* 249 (May 3, 1974): 66.

Wiseman, Paul. "Fabric of a Long Life." *USA Today,* January 3, 2002.

bibliography

selected bibliography

The number of books, manuals, pamphlets, articles, essays, studies, and Internet items verifying lifeforce is limitless. This selected bibliography reflects support for the most crucial and comprehensive aspects of the Hippocrates Program.

Amen, Daniel G. *Healing ADD*. New York: Berkeley Books, 2002.

Atkins, Robert C. *Dr. Atkins' New Diet Revolution*. New York: HarperCollins, 2002.

———. *Dr. Atkins' Nutrition Breakthrough: How to Treat Your Medical Condition Without Drugs*. New York: William Morrow and Company, 1981.

Balch, James F., and Phyllis A. Balch. *Prescription for Nutritional Healing: A Practical A-to-Z Reference to Drug-Free Remedies Using Vitamins, Minerals, Herbs & Food Supplements*. Garden City Park, NY: Avery Publishing Group, 1993.

Barnard, Neal. *Food for Life: How the New Four Food Groups Can Save Your Life*. New York: Harmony Books, 1993.

Bergner, Paul. *The Healing Power of Echinacea & Goldenseal and Other Immune System Herbs*. Rocklin, CA: Prima Publishing, 1997.

Bernay-Roman, Andy. *Deep Feeling, Deep Healing*. Jupiter, FL: Spectrum Healing Press, 2001.

Bloomfield, Harold H., and Robert B. Kory. *The Holistic Way to Health and Happiness*. New York: Fireside, 1978.

Blum, Deborah. *Sex on the Brain: The Biological Differences between Men and Women*. New York: Viking, 1997.

Bolles, Edmund Blair. *Remembering and Forgetting: Inquiries into the Nature of Memory*. New York: Walker and Company, 1988.

Bonar, Ann. *Herbs: A Complete Guide to Their Cultivation and Use*. London: Tiger Books International, 1992.

Bragdon, Allen D., and David Gamon. *Brains That Work a Little Bit Differently: Recent Discoveries about Common Brain Diversities*. New York: Barnes & Noble Books, 2000.

Bricklin, Mark. *Rodale's Encyclopedia of Natural Home Remedies*. Emmaus, PA: Rodale Press, 1991.

Brody, Jane. *Jane Brody's Nutrition Book: A Lifetime Guide to Good Eating for Better Health and Weight Control.* New York: W. W. Norton & Company, 1981.

Buchman, Dian Dincin. *The Complete Book of Water Therapy.* New Canaan, CT: Keats Publishing, 1994.

Campbell, Don. *The Mozart Effect for Children: Awakening Your Child's Mind, Health, and Creativity with Music.* New York: HarperCollins, 2000.

———. *The Mozart Effect: Tapping the Power of Music to Heal the Body, Strengthen the Mind, and Unlock the Creative Spirit.* New York: Avon Books, 1997.

Campbell, T. Colin, and Thomas Campbell. *The China Study: Startling Implications for Diet, Weight Loss and Long-Term Health.* Dallas, TX: Benbella Books, 2006.

Carper, Jean. *Food—Your Miracle Medicine: How Food Can Prevent and Cure over 100 Symptoms and Problems.* New York: HarperCollins, 1993.

Carter, Mildred, and Tammy Weber. *Hand Reflexology: Key to Perfect Health.* Paramus, NJ: Prentice Hall, 2000.

Castleman, Michael. *The Healing Herbs: The Ultimate Guide to the Curative Power of Nature's Medicines.* Emmaus, PA: Rodale Press, 1991.

Chen, Ze-lin, and Mei-fang Chen. *A Comprehensive Guide to Chinese Herbal Medicine.* Edison, NJ: Castle Books, 1999.

Chopra, Deepak. *Ageless Body, Timeless Mind.* New York: Harmony Books, 1993.

———. *Creating Health: Beyond Prevention, Toward Perfection.* Boston: Houghton Mifflin Company, 1987.

Christopher, John R. *School of Natural Healing.* Provo, UT: BiWorld Publishers, 1976.

Claflin, Edward, and the editors of *Prevention* magazine. *Healing Yourself with Food.* Emmaus, PA: Rodale Press, 1995.

Clement, Anna Maria, and Brian R. Clement. *Children: The Ultimate Creation.* West Palm Beach, FL: A. M. Press, 1994.

Clement, Brian R. *Belief: All There Is.* West Palm Beach, FL: Hippocrates Publications, 1991.

———. *Croyances.* Quebec: Les Editions Trustar, 1996.

———. *Exercise: Creating Your Persona.* West Palm Beach, FL: A. M. Press, 1994.

———. *Hippocrates Health Program: A Proven Guide to Healthful Living.* West Palm Beach, FL: Hippocrates Publications, 1989.

———. *Living Foods for Optimum Health: Staying Healthy in an Unhealthy World.* Roseville, CA: Prima Publishing, 1998.

———. *Spirituality in Healing and Life.* West Palm Beach, FL: Hippocrates Publications, 1997.

Clement, Brian R., and Anna Maria Clement. *Relationships: Voyages Through Life.* West Palm Beach, FL: A. M. Press, 1994.

Colgrove, Melba, Harold H. Bloomfield, and Peter McWilliams. *How to Survive the Loss of Love.* Los Angeles: Prelude Press, 1991.

Cox, Peter. *You Don't Need Meat.* New York: Thomas Dunne Books, 2002.

Creff, Albert-François, and Robert Wernick. *Dr. Creff's 1-2-3 Sports Diet.* New York: Coward, McCann & Geoghan, 1979.

Dalai Lama and Howard C. Cutler. *The Art of Happiness.* New York: Riverhead Books, 1998.

Deacon, Terrence W. *The Symbolic Species: The Co-evolution of Language and the Brain*. New York: W. W. Norton & Company, 1997.

Dharma Singh Khalsa with Cameron Stauth. *Brain Longevity*. New York: Warner Books, 1997.

Diamond, Harvey. *Fit for Life: A New Beginning—The Ultimate Diet and Health Plan*. New York: Kensington Books, 2000.

Diamond, Harvey, and Marilyn Diamond. *Fit for Life: The Natural Body Cycle, Permanent Weight Loss Plan That Proves It's Not What You Eat, but When and How*. New York: Warner Books, 1985.

Disease Prevention and Treatment. Hollywood, FL: Life Extension Foundation, 2003.

Dodt, Colleen K. *The Essential Oils Book: Creating Personal Blends for Mind & Body*. Pownal, VT: Storey Communications, 1996.

Dossey, Larry. *Healing Words: The Power of Prayer and the Practice of Medicine*. San Francisco: HarperSanFrancisco, 1993.

Duke, James A. *Dr. Duke's Essential Herbs*. Emmaus, PA: Rodale, 1999.

———. *The Green Pharmacy*. Emmaus, PA: Rodale, 1997.

Durrell, Gerald. *My Family and Other Animals*. New York: Penguin Books, 1976.

Evans, Mark. *Natural Home Remedies: Safe, Effective and Traditional Treatments for Common Ailments*. New York: Anness Publishing, 1996.

Farmilant, Eunice. *The Natural Foods Sweet Tooth Cookbook*. New York: Pyramid Books, 1975.

Finley, Anita, and Bill Finley. *Live to Be 100 Plus: Chart Your Way to a Longer Life*. Boca Raton, FL: Senior Life Press, 1992.

Fischer-Rizzi, Susanne. *Medicine of the Earth: Legends, Recipes, and Cultivation of Healing Plants*. Portland, OR: Rudra Press, 1996.

Fitzgerald, Randall. *The Hundred-Year Lie: How Food and Medicine Are Destroying Your Health*. New York: Penguin/Dutton, 2006.

Forni, P. M. *Choosing Civility: The Twenty-five Rules of Considerate Conduct*. New York: St. Martin's Press, 2002.

Foster, Steven. *101 Medicinal Herbs: An Illustrated Guide*. Loveland, CO: Interweave Press, 1998.

Fraser, Linda. *Classic Vegetarian Cooking*. London: Barnes & Noble Books, 2001.

Fuhrman, Joel. *Eat to Live: The Revolutionary Formula for Fast and Sustained Weight Loss*. Boston: Little, Brown and Company, 2003.

Glynn, Ian. *An Anatomy of Thought: The Origin and Machinery of the Mind*. New York: Oxford University Press, 1999.

Goleman, Daniel. *Emotional Intelligence*. New York: Bantam Books, 1995.

Gosselin, Robert E., Harold C. Hodge, Roger P. Smith, and Marion N. Gleason. *Clinical Toxicology of Commercial Products*. Baltimore: Williams & Wilkins, 1977.

Haas, Robert. *Eat to Win*. New York: Signet, 1983.

———. *Permanent Remissions: Life Extending Diet Strategies That Can Help Prevent and Reverse Cancer, Heart Disease, Diabetes, and Osteoporosis*. New York: Pocket Books, 1997.

Haber, David. *Health Promotion and Aging: Implications for the Health Professions*. New York: Springer Publishing Company, 1999.

The Harvard Medical School Health Letter Book. Cambridge, MA: Harvard University Press, 1981.

Hill, Napoleon, and Michael J. Ritt Jr. *Napoleon Hill's Keys to Positive Thinking: 10 Steps to Health, Wealth and Success*. New York: Dutton, 1998.

Hobson, J. Allan. *The Chemistry of Conscious States: How the Brain Changes Its Mind*. New York: Little, Brown and Company, 1994.

Hogshead, Nancy, and Gerald S. Cousens. *Asthma and Exercise*. New York: Henry Holt and Company, 1990.

Holford, Patrick, and Hyla Cass. *Natural Highs: Increase Your Energy; Sharpen Your Mind; Improve Your Mood; Relax and Beat Stress with Legal, Natural and Healthy Mind-Altering Substances*. London: Judy Piatkus Publishers, 2001.

Howard, Pierce J. *The Owner's Manual for the Brain: Everyday Applications from Mind-Brain Research*. Austin, TX: Leornian Press, 1994.

Hutton, Ginger. *Reflections: Thoughts on Love and Living*. Phoenix, AZ: Arizona Republic, 1980.

Jensen, Bernard. *Dr. Jensen's Juicing Therapy: Nature's Way to Better Health and a Longer Life*. Los Angeles: Keats Publishing, 2000.

LeDoux, Joseph. *The Emotional Brain*. New York: Touchstone, 1996.

Lerner, Harriet. *The Dance of Anger: A Woman's Guide to Changing the Patterns of Intimate Relationships*. New York: Perennial Library, 1989.

Levine, Stephen. *Healing Into Life and Death*. New York: Anchor Books, 1977.

Lipschitz, David A. *Breaking the Rules of Aging*. Washington, DC: Lifeline Press, 2002.

Lipton, Bruce. *The Biology of Belief*. Santa Rosa, CA: Elite Books, 2005.

Little, Paul E. *Know Why You Believe*. Wheaton, IL: Victor Books, 1973.

Lockie, Andrew, and Nicola Geddes. *Complete Guide to Homeopathy*. New York: DK Publishing, 2000.

Lowe, Carl, James W. Nechas, and the editors of *Prevention* magazine. *Whole Body Healing: Natural Healing with Movement, Exercise, Massage and Other Drug-Free Methods*. Emmaus, PA: Rodale Press, 1983.

Mamonov, Valery. *Control for Life Extension: A Personalized Holistic Approach*. Rome, ME: Long Life Press, 2001.

Marshall, John, with Heather Barbash. *The Sports Doctor's Fitness Book for Women*. New York: Delacorte Press, 1981.

Messina, Virginia, and Mark Messina. *The Vegetarian Way: Total Health for You and Your Family*. New York: Crown, 1996.

Mindell, Earl R. *Earl Mindell's Food as Medicine: What You Can Eat to Help Prevent Everything from Colds to Heart Disease to Cancer*. New York: Fireside (Simon & Schuster), 1994.

Navarra, Tova, and Myron A. Lipkowitz. *Encyclopedia of Vitamins, Minerals and Supplements*. New York: Facts on File, 1996.

Naylor, Nicola. *Discover Essential Oils*. Berkeley, CA: Ulysses Press, 1998.

Nirenberg, Jesse S. *Getting Through to People*. Englewood Cliffs, NJ: Prentice Hall, 1963.

Northrup, Christiane. *Women's Bodies, Women's Wisdom: Creating Physical and Emotional Health and Healing*. New York: Bantam Books, 1998.

Ohno, Yoshitaka. *A Guide to Achieving Better Health and Aging.* Willoughby, OH: Ohno Institute on Water and Health, undated.

Passwater, Richard A. *The Longevity Factor: Chromium Picolinate.* New Canaan, CT: Keats Publishing, 1993.

Peck, M. Scott. *The Road Less Traveled: A New Psychology of Love, Traditional Values and Spiritual Growth.* New York: Touchstone, 1978.

Peikin, Steven R. *The Feel Full Diet: The Medically Proven, Nutritionally Sound Weight Loss Program That Stimulates the Release of Your Secret Anti-hunger Mechanism.* New York: Atheneum, 1987.

Physician's Guide to Remedies and Cures. Greenwich, CT: Boardroom, Inc., 1999.

Pritikin, Nathan. *The Pritikin Weight Loss Manual.* New York: Grosset & Dunlap, 1981.

Ratey, John J. *A User's Guide to the Brain: Perception, Attention, and the Four Theaters of the Brain.* New York: Vintage Books, 2001.

Rath, Matthias. *Why Animals Don't Get Heart Attacks . . . But People Do.* Fremont, CA: MR Publishing, 2003.

Reich, Charles A. *The Greening of America.* New York: Random House, 1970.

Reid, Daniel P. *Chinese Herbal Medicine.* Boston: Shambhala Publications, 1999.

———. *The Complete Book of Chinese Health and Healing.* Boston: Shambhala Publications, 1995.

Reinhard, Tonia. *The Vitamin Sourcebook.* Los Angeles: Lowell House, 1998.

Restak, Richard. *Mozart's Brain and the Fighter Pilot: Unleashing Your Brain's Potential.* New York: Harmony Books, 2001.

Reuben, David. *Everything You Always Wanted to Know about Nutrition.* New York: Avon Books, 1978.

Rister, Robert. *Japanese Herbal Medicine: The Healing Art of Kampo.* Garden City Park, NY: Avery Publishing Group, 1999.

Robbins, John. *Diet for a New America: How Your Food Choices Affect Your Health, Happiness and the Future of Life on Earth.* Walpole, NH: Stillpoint Publishing, 1987.

———. *Reclaiming Our Health: Exploding the Medical Myth and Embracing the Source of True Healing.* Tiburon, CA: H. J. Kramer, 1996.

Robbins, William. *The American Food Scandal.* New York: William Morrow and Company, 1974.

Robertson, Ian H. *Mind Sculpture: Unlocking Your Brain's Untapped Potential.* New York: Fromm International, 2000.

Rodale, Robert, ed. *The Basic Book of Organic Gardening.* New York: Ballantine Books, 1971.

Rondberg, Terry A. *Chiropractic First: The Fastest Growing Healthcare Choice—Before Drugs or Surgery.* Chandler, AZ: Chiropractic Journal, 1996.

Rose, Barry, and Christina Scott Moncrief. *Homeopathy for Women.* London: Collins & Brown, 1998.

Rosenfeld, Isadore. *The Complete Medical Exam.* New York: Avon Books, 1978.

Rosner, Fred, ed. and trans. *Maimonides: Medical Writings.* Multivolume series. Haifa, Israel: Maimonides Research Institute, ongoing.

Schiller, Carol, and David Schiller. *500 Formulas for Aromatherapy: Mixing Essential Oils for Every Use.* New York: Sterling Publishing, 1994.

Schnaubelt, Kurt. *Medical Aromatherapy: Healing with Essential Oils*. Berkeley, CA: Frog, 1999.

Sears, Barry, with Bill Lawren. *Enter the Zone: A Dietary Road Map*. New York: Regan Books, 1995.

Segal, Jeanne. *Raising Your Emotional Intelligence*. New York: Henry Holt and Company, 1997.

Serrentino, Joe. *How Natural Remedies Work: Vitamins, Minerals, Nutrients, Homeopathic and Naturopathic Remedies*. Point Roberts, WA: Hartley & Marks, 1991.

Siegel, Bernie S. *Love, Medicine and Miracles: Lessons Learned about Self-Healing from a Surgeon's Experience with Exceptional Patients*. New York: Harper & Row, 1987.

Simonton, O. Carl, Stephanie Mathews-Simonton, and James L. Creighton. *Getting Well Again*. New York: Bantam Books, 1992.

Smith, Adam. *Powers of Mind*. New York: Random House, 1975.

Smith, Jeffrey M. *Seeds of Deception: Exposing Industry and Government Lies about the Safety of the Genetically Engineered Foods You're Eating*. Fairfield, IA: Yes! Books, 2003.

Snow, Kimberly. *In Buddha's Kitchen*. Boston: Shambhala Publications, 2003.

Staudacher, Carol. *Men and Grief*. Oakland, CA: New Harbinger Publications, 1991.

Stein, Laura. *The Bloomingdale's Eat Healthy Diet*. New York: St. Martin's Press, 1986.

Steiner, Claude, with Paul Perry. *Achieving Emotional Literacy: A Personal Program to Increase Your Emotional Intelligence*. New York: Avon Books, 1997.

Stillerman, Elaine. *The Encyclopedia of Bodywork*. New York: Facts on File, 1996.

Stone, Irwin. *The Healing Factor: "Vitamin C" Against Disease*. New York: Grosset & Dunlap, 1972.

Thayer, Robert E. *The Origin of Everyday Moods: Managing Energy, Tension, and Stress*. New York: Oxford University Press, 1996.

Thomas, Peggy. *Medicines from Nature*. New York: Twenty-First Century Books, 1997.

Tisserand, Robert B. *The Art of Aromatherapy: The Healing and Beautifying Properties of the Essential Oils of Flowers and Herbs*. Rochester, VT: Healing Arts Press, 1977.

Ursell, Amanda. *Vitamins and Minerals Handbook: Nature-Inspired Supplements for Optimal Health and Vitality*. New York: Dorling Kindersley, 2001.

Vertosick, Frank, Jr. *When the Air Hits Your Brain: Tales of Neurosurgery*. New York: W. W. Norton & Company, 1996.

Walker, N. W. *The Vegetarian Guide to Diet & Salad*. Phoenix, AZ: Norwalk Press, 1986.

Weber, George. *Protecting Your Health with Probiotics: The Friendly Bacteria*. Green Bay, WI: IMPAKT Communications, 2001.

Wood, Garth. *The Myth of Neurosis: Overcoming the Illness Excuse*. New York: Harper & Row, 1986.

Wright, Jane Riddle. *Diagnosis: Cancer—Prognosis: Life*. Huntsville, AL: Albright & Co., 1985.

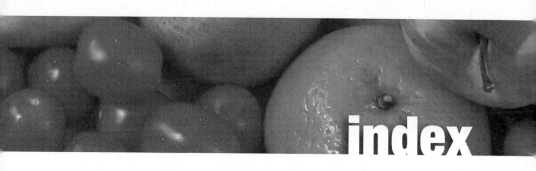

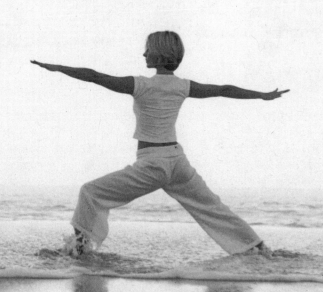

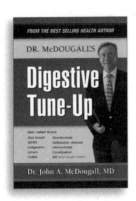
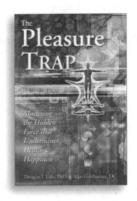
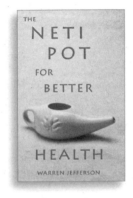
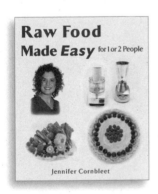
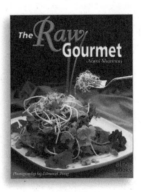
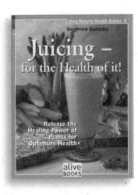